T0200395

ADVANCES IN

Family Practice Nursing

Editor-in-Chief
Geri C. Reeves, PhD, APRN, FNP-BC

Associate Editors
Sharon L. Holley, DNP, CNM, FACNM

Linda J. Keilman, DNP, GNP-BC, FAANP

Imelda Reyes, DNP, MPH, APRN, CPNP-PC, FNP-BC, FAANP

ELSEVIER

PHILADELPHIA   LONDON   TORONTO   MONTREAL   SYDNEY   TOKYO

Editor: Kerry Holland
Developmental Editor: Axell Purificacion

Reprints: For copies of 100 or more of articles in this publication, please contact the Commercial Reprints Department, Elsevier Inc., 360 Park Avenue South, New York, NY 10010-1710. Tel: (212) 633-3812; Fax: (212) 462-1935; E-mail: reprints@elsevier.com.

Printed in the United States of America.

Editorial Office:
Elsevier
1600 John F. Kennedy Blvd,
Suite 1800
Philadelphia, PA 19103-2899

International Standard Serial Number: 2589-4722
International Standard Book Number: 978-0-323-81100-2

CONTRIBUTORS

BETH A. AMMERMAN, DNP, FNP-BC, Clinical Assistant Professor and Family Nurse Practitioner, University of Michigan School of Nursing, Ann Arbor, Michigan

LINDSEY BAKSH, DNP, WHNP-BC, Instructor in Nursing, Vanderbilt University School of Nursing, Nashville, Tennessee

ERIN DeBRUYN, DNP, APRN, WHNP-BC, Instructor of Nursing, Vanderbilt University School of Nursing, Nashville, Tennessee

JESSE CASAUBON, DO, Department of Surgery, University of Massachusetts Medical School–Baystate, Springfield, Massachusetts

PATRICK C. CRANE, DNP, RN, AGPCNP-BC, Michigan State University, College of Nursing, East Lansing, Michigan

LACEY CROSS, MSN, FNP-BC, Instructor, Vanderbilt University School of Nursing, Nashville, Tennessee

KATHERINE DONTJE, PhD, FNP-BC, FAANP, Michigan State University, College of Nursing, East Lansing, Michigan

ELIZABETH GALIK, PhD, CRNP, FAAN, FAANP, Professor, University of Maryland School of Nursing, Baltimore, Maryland

VANESSA GRAFTON, MSN, CNM, Carle Foundation Hospital, Urbana, Illinois

QUEEN HENRY-OKAFOR, PhD, FNP-BC, PMHNP-BC, Assistant Professor, Vanderbilt University School of Nursing, Nashville, Tennessee

SHARON L. HOLLEY, DNP, CNM, FACNM, Chief, Division of Midwifery and Community Health, Associate Professor, Department of Obstetrics and Gynecology, University of Massachusetts Medical School–Baystate, Baystate Medical Center, Springfield, Massachusetts

MADISON N. IRWIN, PharmD, Department of Pharmacy, Michigan Medicine, University of Michigan College of Pharmacy, Ann Arbor, Michigan

LINDA J. KEILMAN, DNP, GNP-BC, FAANP, Associate Professor, Gerontology Population Content Expert, Gerontological Nurse Practitioner, Michigan State University, College of Nursing, East Lansing, Michigan

DANIELLE LIPOFF, DO, MS, Department of Surgery, University of Massachusetts Medical School–Baystate, Springfield, Massachusetts

ERINN M. LOUTTIT, MSN, FNP-BC, Pediatric Palliative Care, Michigan Medicine, Ann Arbor, Michigan

HEATHER LOVE, MD, MPH, Department of Obstetrics and Gynecology, University of Massachusetts Medical School–Baystate, Springfield, Massachusetts

HOLLY MASON, MD, Department of Surgery, University of Massachusetts Medical School–Baystate, Springfield, Massachusetts

GINNY MOORE, DNP, WHNP-BC, Associate Professor and WHNP Academic Director, Vanderbilt University School of Nursing, Nashville, Tennessee

ELIZABETH MUÑOZ, MSN, CNM, Carle Foundation Hospital, University of Illinois Chicago, Vanderbilt University School of Nursing, Urbana, Illinois

NINA GANESH NANDISH, AGPCNP-BC, Adult and Gerontology Primary Care Nurse Practitioner, Medicine, Livonia, Michigan

NILAN NANDISH, Research Assistant, Medicine, Livonia, Michigan

SHIVA NIAKAN, DO, Department of Obstetrics and Gynecology, University of Massachusetts Medical School–Baystate, Springfield, Massachusetts

MELISSA OTT, DNP, PMHNP-BC, FNP-BC, Instructor of Nursing, Vanderbilt University School of Nursing, Nashville, Tennessee

SHAUNNA PARKER, MSN, WHNP-BC, Instructor in Nursing, Vanderbilt University School of Nursing, Nashville, Tennessee

ELIZABETH A. PASTERNAK, MS-PREP, BSN, Pediatric Palliative Care, Michigan Medicine, Ann Arbor, Michigan

MARY LAUREN PFIEFFER, DNP, FNP-BC, Assistant Professor, Vanderbilt University School of Nursing, Nashville, Tennessee

BREIA REED, MS, Medical Student, Meharry Medical School, Nashville, Tennessee

GERI C. REEVES, PhD, APRN, FNP-BC, Associate Professor, Family Nurse Practitioner Program, Vanderbilt University School of Nursing, Nashville, Tennessee

IMELDA REYES, DNP, MPH, APRN, CPNP-PC, FNP-BC, FAANP, Associate Clinical Professor, Pediatric Primary Care NP Specialty Coordinator, DNP Population Health Track Coordinator, Emory University, Nell Hodgson Woodruff School of Nursing, Atlanta, Georgia

SHELZA RIVAS, DNP, WHNP-BC, AGPCNP-BC, Instructor in Nursing, Vanderbilt University School of Nursing, Nashville, Tennessee

ELLEN SOLIS, DNP, CNM, Carle Foundation Hospital, University of Illinois Chicago, Urbana, Illinois

JESSICA L. SPRUIT, DNP, CPNP-AC, Wayne State University College of Nursing, Michigan Medicine Pediatric Palliative Care, Detroit, Michigan

JULIA M. STEED, PhD, APRN, FNP-BC, CTTS, Assistant Professor, Vanderbilt University School of Nursing, Nashville, Tennessee

TERESA WHITED, DNP, APRN, CPNP-PC, Associate Dean of Academic Programs, Clinical Associate Professor, University of Arkansas for Medical Sciences, College of Nursing, Little Rock, Arkansas

TERI MOSER WOO, PhD, ARNP, CPNP-PC, CNL, FAANP, Professor and Director of Nursing, Saint Martin's University, Lacey, Washington; ARNP at Convenience Care by Woodcreek Pediatrics – Mary Bridge Children's, Puyallup, Washington

JENNIFER J. WRIGHT, MS, CPNP-PC, Pediatric Palliative Care, Michigan Medicine, Ann Arbor, Michigan

Obstructive Sleep Apnea in Older Adults: Diagnosis and Management
Nina Ganesh Nandish, Nilan Nandish

Assessment and Management of Constipation in Older Adults
Linda J. Keilman and Katherine Dontje

Genitourinary Syndrome of Menopause: Screening and Treatment

Queen Henry-Okafor, Erin DeBruyn, Melissa Ott, and
Ginny Moore

Best Practices in Breast Health and Breast Cancer Screening

Shiva Niakan, Heather Love, Danielle Lipoff, Jesse Casaubon,
and Holly Mason

Smoking and Maternal Health: Evidence that Female Infertility Can Be Attributed to Smoking and Improved with Smoking Cessation
Julia M. Steed, Shaunna Parker, and Breia Reed

Opioid Use Disorder Screening for Women Across the Lifespan
Ginny Moore, Lindsey Baksh, Shaunna Parker, and
Shelza Rivas

Pediatrics

Pediatric Pharmacology Update
Teri Moser Woo

New and Reemerging Infectious Diseases in Pediatrics
Teresa Whited

Pain Management in Pediatrics

Elizabeth A. Pasternak, Erinn M. Louttit, Jennifer J. Wright,
Madison N. Irwin, and Jessica L. Spruit

PREFACE

Primary Care During COVID-19 and Beyond

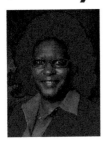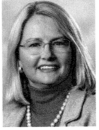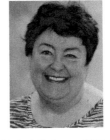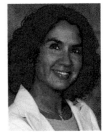

Geri C. Reeves, PhD, APRN, FNP-BC

Sharon L. Holley, DNP, CNM, FACNM

Linda J. Keilman, DNP, GNP-BC, FAANP

Imelda Reyes, DNP, MPH, APRN, CPNP-PC, FNP-BC, FAANP

Editors

The novel coronavirus outbreak was declared a public health emergency of international concern on January 30, 2020. As of this writing, on October 19, 2020, there have been 39,944,882 confirmed cases of COVID-19 worldwide with 1,111,998 confirmed deaths globally.[1] In the United States, 8,393,773 people have contracted the virus, and there are 224,824 confirmed deaths.[2] These staggering statistics represent the worst pandemic in modern times. The current COVID-19 pandemic taught us important lessons about how primary care (PC) can respond during a pandemic. The role of PC as the first point of contact to the health care system should not change during a pandemic. As the first line of defense, PC has the potential to reinforce critical public health messages, help patients manage infections at home, and identify those in need of inpatient care.[3] Done well, this can reduce the spread of infection and protect hospitals from being overwhelmed.[3] Yet, the realities of a fragmented health care system became evident during the COVID-19 pandemic.

PC practices can adapt and continue to reinvent themselves during a pandemic using the Center for Disease Control and Prevention's pandemic framework–recommended actions. The core principle is protecting clinicians, staff, and patients while remaining available and connected to meet patient needs.[3] Yet, in response to the COVID-19 pandemic, practices struggled to rapidly adapt to demands. Testing was not available, and contact tracing

https://doi.org/10.1016/j.yfpn.2021.02.006

2589-420X/21/© 2021 Published by Elsevier Inc.

was not possible. As the pandemic spread, many practices converted to virtual care using telehealth.[3,4] Though not commonly tested in disaster settings, telemedicine was a crucial component of the medical response to COVID-19 by reducing demand on strained health care infrastructure and enabling health care needs to be met at home while reducing exposure for patients and health care staff. In fact, the widespread adoption of telemedicine associated with the COVID-19 pandemic was unprecedented and will likely have a significant and durable impact on health care delivery.[4]

The current pandemic also made the need for access to affordable care to all painfully clear. Well-known social determinants of health, such as educational attainment, occupation, place of residence, access to affordable and healthy food, and race or ethnicity, are key factors that influence one's ability to safely weather a global pandemic of a highly infectious disease.[5] What is more, approximately half of Americans receive health coverage through their employer, and with high numbers filing for unemployment insurance, millions find themselves without health insurance during the largest pandemic in a century.[6] Failure to receive testing and treatment because of cost harms everyone by prolonging the pandemic, increasing its morbidity and mortality, and worsening its economic impact.[6]

To address numerous issues raised by COVID-19, the US Congress has passed 2 significant pieces of legislation. The Families First Coronavirus Response Act requires all private insurers, Medicare, Medicare Advantage, and Medicaid to cover COVID-19 testing and eliminate all cost sharing. It also appropriated $1 billion for the Public Health and Social Services Emergency Fund to cover testing for uninsured individuals under state Medicaid plans. These laws provide critical assistance. However, additional policies are needed to ensure that Americans can continue to access affordable care as the crisis continues and beyond.[6] Policymakers and payers must ensure that funding and policies allow PC to transform and adapt to COVID-19's impact on our nation's health care system. The health and well-being of all Americans depend on it. As PC providers, you are uniquely qualified to advocate for policies and funding that protect clinicians, staff, and patients. We must continue to call on our nation's leaders to address the needs of PC during the current pandemic and beyond.

To further support PC practices in providing health care needs, you will find, in this issue of *Advances in Family Practice Nursing*, information on infectious disease prevention, older adults and driving cessation, diagnosis and management of obstructive sleep apnea, management of constipation in older adults, dementia, evidence-based care for pregnancy complicated by obesity, smoking and maternal health, screening and treatment for genitourinary syndrome of menopause, updates on Pap smear guidelines, mammogram screening, pharmacology in pediatrics, and sports medicine. We trust that this issue will provide timely and relevant information that will support the management of your patients.

Geri C. Reeves, PhD, APRN, FNP-BC
Vanderbilt University
360 Frist Hall
Nashville, TN 37240, USA

E-mail address: geri.reeves@Vanderbilt.Edu

Sharon L. Holley, DNP, CNM, FACNM
Baystate Medical Center
689 Chestnut Street
Springfield, MA 01199, USA

E-mail address: Sharon.holley@baystatehealth.org

Linda J. Keilman, DNP, GNP-BC, FAANP
Michigan State University
College of Nursing
1355 Bogue Street
A126 Life Science Building
East Lansing, MI 48824-1317, USA

E-mail address: keilman@msu.edu

Imelda Reyes, DNP, MPH, APRN, CPNP-PC, FNP-BC, FAANP
Emory University
Nell Hodgson Woodruff School of Nursing
1520 Clifton Road, Suite 432
Atlanta, GA 30322, USA

E-mail address: ireyes@emory.edu

References

1 World Health Organization. Coronavirus disease (COVID-19) pandemic. Available at: https://www.who.int/emergencies/diseases/novel-coronavirus-2019. Accessed October 6, 2020.
2 Centers for Disease Control and Prevention. United States COVID-19 cases and deaths by state. Available at: https://covid.cdc.gov/covid-data-tracker/#cases_casesinlast7days. Accessed October 6, 2020.
3 Krist AH, DeVoe JE, Cheng A, et al. Redesigning primary care to address the COVID-19 pandemic during the pandemic. Ann Fam Med 2020;18(4):349–54.
4 Ramaswamy A, Yu M, Drangsholt S, et al. Patient satisfaction with telemedicine during the COVID-19 pandemic: retrospective cohort study. J Med Internet Res 2020;22(9):e20786.
5 Wolfson JA, Leung CW. An opportunity to emphasize equity, social determinants, and prevention in primary care. Ann Fam Med 2020;18:290–1.
6 King JS. Covid-19 and the need for health care reform. New Engl J Med 2020;328(26):e104.

Adult/Geriatric

Older Adults and Driving Cessation
Knowing When and How to Approach the Conversation

Beth A. Ammerman, DNP, FNP-BC

University of Michigan School of Nursing, 400 North Ingalls, Room 3179, Ann Arbor, MI 48901, USA

Keywords

- Older adult driving • Difficult discussions • Aging changes • Communication
- Mobility

Key points

- Driving is a form of independence that most human beings cherish and anticipate with great excitement when reaching the age of licensure.
- With normal aging, there are mental and physical changes that occur that make safe driving more difficult.
- Older adult driving retirement must be a conversation between the patient and health care professional yearly, at a minimum, and with any change of condition.
- Health care professionals need to understand the value and purpose of difficult conversations and gain experience in delivering information the patient may not want to hear.
- Health care professionals and their primary care staff need to know the community resources available for older adults as they are transitioning into driving retirement and what they will consider a loss of independence.

INTRODUCTION

Mr P is a 77-year-old widowed man who, despite his advanced metastatic cancer, had remained very active until recently. He never really enjoyed cooking for himself, so he really looked forward to eating and socializing with friends at a local restaurant. His days included running errands, meeting friends, getting his grandchildren on the school bus, attending frequent health care appointments, and participating in the local ballroom dancing club. His driving

E-mail address: bammerma@umich.edu

https://doi.org/10.1016/j.yfpn.2021.02.003
2589-420X/21/© 2021 Elsevier Inc. All rights reserved.

afforded him the independence to do the things he wanted and to care for himself independently, without relying on others. As his cancer progressed and he became physically weaker, walking for Mr P became increasingly difficult, although he remained mentally sharp. He was struggling to pump gas, ambulate on his own, and could no longer dance. He had 3 minor fender benders in the past month and his daughter noticed he struggled to keep the car between the lines on the road. Upon discharge from his most recent hospitalization, he asked his doctor when he could drive again. It was obvious to his family that he was no longer safe on the roads. Mr P's physician told Mr P's daughter to ride with him and she could decide when he was recovered enough to drive again. Mr P's children left the car in the garage but hid his keys.

Mrs R, an 80-year-old married woman, presented to her primary care office for a routine yearly checkup. While in the room, her husband mentioned to the health care provider (HCP) that she seemed more forgetful over the past year. During the interview, Mrs R relied on her husband to answer most of the questions for her. As a retired school bus driver, Mrs R had always loved to drive her own car, yet over the past few years, she had become increasingly reliant on her husband to navigate for her. He stated it was not his place to stop her from driving, but he was afraid for her and for others on the road. He will only let her drive if he was in the car because she got lost and frequently made turns in front of other cars.

Mrs G is a 58-year-old petite woman with progressive multiple sclerosis and worsening weakness in the legs. She lives alone, but her son lives nearby. She struggles to ambulate, even with a walker. She would drive about town daily, going through drive-through restaurants, banking from the car, driving by friends' houses, and picking up groceries daily. Her son knew that she could not feel which foot was on the gas and brake pedals, but he did not want to rob her of her freedom. She got very angry every time he mentioned maybe she should not be driving any longer, so he gave up.

These 3 scenarios represent actual patient situations that depict reality for many older drivers and concerned families. They also represent times when an HCP had an opportunity to assist struggling older drivers and their families make a sound plan for retirement from driving.

The privilege and freedom to drive

Driving is a privilege most often earned during the teenage years. Driving represents freedom, independence, and competence and provides an autonomous way for people to get where they want to go and when they want to go. However, it is widely recognized that driving requires high level skills like keen eyesight, quick reflexes, and advanced decision-making to safely maneuver a car through changing road conditions [1]. There is an established initiation process for teens to become licensed drivers including:

- Participation in a drivers' education course
- Mandatory driving practice in different road conditions
- Passing both a written examination and a supervised road driving test

• Fees for driving education course, testing, permit, licensing, and insurance

Although teenagers may exhibit the physical and cognitive abilities needed to drive early on, they still must wait until a predetermined age (usually 16 or 17 years old) before they can drive legally. Inauguration of driving is therefore both ability and age dependent.

Conversely, the cessation of driving is highly variable. There is no predetermined age nor mandatory testing that dictates when an older adult must retire their driving privileges. There are age-related health changes that can negatively impact driving ability. Decreased eyesight, stiffened joints, weakened gait, decreased hearing, increased confusion, decreasing cognitive function, and slowed response time can all make driving increasingly more difficult. Because the loss of driving rights represents the loss of independence, there is a risk that older adults will continue to drive after they are no longer safely able to maneuver a vehicle. When safety is a concern, it becomes necessary to talk about driving cessation or retirement. This discussion can be very difficult and is often emotionally charged. It is frequently not the aging driver, but the aging driver's family or close friends, who turn to the HCP for help. Although it is logical that a trusted HCP would assess and assist in this transition from driving to nondriving, many HCP feel ill-prepared to handle this discussion and uncomfortable making the recommendations regarding the cessation of driving. This article explores the background and addresses:

• Driving impairment in older adults
• Steps for HCP to facilitate an effective driving retirement discussion
• Resources for the HCP to use during a dedicated appointment to help a patient plan for driving retirement

BACKGROUND

Today there are more mature licensed drivers than in previous generations. In 2017, there were approximately twice as many drivers greater than age 65 years than there were in 1994 [2]. As people live longer and remain healthier, their driving years are extended. Statistics show that nearly 85% of people aged 70 to 84 years old, and nearly 61% of people over 85 years of age still hold a driver's license [3]. By 2050, it is predicted that one in 4 US drivers will be over the age of 65 years [4]. In many ways, healthy and able older adults tend to exhibit safer driving habits than younger people; they wear their seatbelts, limit driving under poor conditions, speed less, are less likely to drive after drinking alcohol, and are less likely to use cell phones or text while driving [5]. However, as the age of older drivers increases, so do motor vehicle accidents and fatalities. Drivers over 75 years of age are at a higher risk for fatalities than younger drivers owing to greater fragility, resulting in more severe injuries [6]. Eventually, it becomes evident that the road to driving must end. Planning ahead is a necessity and the HCP can help patients to plan for this upcoming loss in a positive manner.

ASSESSMENT OF DRIVING ABILITY
Routine assessment for driving retirement
The best time to initiate a "when to retire driving" conversation is before there are any impairments. As an HCP, these conversations are necessary and can be initiated in multiple thoughtful ways, preserving the dignity of the older adult. Ideally, a best practice is to establish a routine of introducing the subject of driving retirement with all older patients, making it a normal part of the health assessment. The subject should be initiated well before any issues or red flags arise. Asking simply, "At some point you will most likely stop driving a car. When do you see yourself retiring from driving?" might be a neutral question to break into the conversation. In addition, providing older adults and their families with a list of red flags can help them to monitor an older adult's driving and help them to know when to alert the HCP and inform them if any changes occur. Red flags for driving impairment are included in Box 1.

Planning for driving retirement
During a routine health care appointment, time is usually spent on the presenting health concern. Often the subject of one's driving is brought up near the end of a visit, often by the driver's relative, and often catches the HCP off guard. Retirement from employment often takes years of planning and many discussions. When the discussion or planning is about retiring from driving, it should not be a quick discussion held at the end of a regularly scheduled appointment.

Difficult conversations should have dedicated time set aside to plan for a multiphasic approach. It is best practice to discuss the subject while the patient is healthy, has the capacity to make safe decisions, and retirement from driving is not immediate. This conversation should involve the older adult in transparent communication, identifying the older adult's timeline and plan for retirement from driving. Of course, older adult drivers and their HCP do not always

---

Box 1: Red flags for older adult driver impairment [7,8]
Forgetting where they are in familiar places
Motor vehicle accidents: crashes or near crashes
Disregarding stop signs and traffic signals
Reaction time is slowed
Unable to reach the pedals and/or see over the steering wheel
Unable to turn head appropriately to see out all windows/mirrors
Getting angry at other drivers
Having trouble judging distances
Forgetting or ignoring driving basics
Progressive severe chronic debilitating disease
Unable to see well at night or day

get ideal situations. Generally, a sudden illness or injury occurs, leaving the patient unable to drive, which becomes an emotionally charged conversation, especially if the patient has a strong desire to continue to drive. The conversation should really occur over a period of time with a series of conversations, planning, and checkins [9].

Betz and colleagues [10] noted that HCPs are trusted and viewed as authority figures and patients listen to them. This makes the HCP the ideal person to initiate this difficult conversation. Although it seems logical the HCP is the natural choice for this discussion, many HCPs feel unprepared to handle this uncomfortable conversation [5]. Fewer than 6% of older drivers report having a discussion with their HCP about when they plan to stop driving [10]. HCPs reported talking about driving cessation with their oldest old drivers and not with younger older drivers [11].

Older adults are more apt to respond well to planning conversations when they are initiated by their HCP. Betz and colleagues also found that more than 80% of patients believed that planning ahead could make the emotional transition much easier once they retired from driving. Betz and colleagues also found that older adult patients who planned out driving cessation thought they would be closer to retirement from driving [12] and within 5 to 7 years of death [13]. Although many studies show that drivers would rather hear about their poor, unsafe driving from a spouse or family member first, they still felt their HCPs were knowledgeable and very trusted to discuss driving cessation [11].

The conversation

Difficult conversations, especially one where an older adult driving privilege is at stake, are not comfortable for the patient, families, or HCP. Conversations about an older adult ability to drive safely often are initiated at inopportune times such as when:

- There is an immediate health reason to at least temporarily quit driving;
- There is no time scheduled for the discussion; and
- The older adult was unaware of the concern, all of which can create an even more uncomfortable setting for this difficult discussion.

Most often the conversation is initiated because the patient is having symptoms and cessation of driving is more likely soon. Generally, it is not the older adult's decision to quit driving; in fact, the older adult often strongly desires to continue driving, making this an emotionally charged discussion. Concerns about an older adult driving might be initiated by a family member or close friend, and not by the patient. Owing to patient health privacy guidelines, the moment can be even more awkward. Often a spouse, a child, a close friend, or another family member may express concern over changes they've noticed in the older adult's driving. From this perspective, it is best to approach the older adult directly and privately with questions about their driving. Sometimes the family or friend may have privately contacted the HCP about the driving concern. It might be best not to tell the older adult if a concern was raised by their family or friend, so as not to alienate them from their family and friends if driving is suddenly retired. In a difficult conversation where older adult driving and independence are at stake, someone is going to be the bad guy, and it most likely could be the HCP. Handling the conversation with decorum and respecting the older adult's dignity are essential. It is best not to alienate the older adult from their support system. Sometimes, the older adult might express concerns about their own driving. If the older adult patient brings up the subject, or if the family or friend brings it up in the patient's presence, there is more transparency and freedom to ask questions openly about driving behaviors.

ASSESSMENT OF DRIVING IMPAIRMENT

If the conversation is directly with the older adult, the focus should be on them; the HCP should be supportive and understanding. The HCP can encourage the older adult to make an eye appointment, bring in their medications for review, and set-up a physical examination appointment. During the conversation, the HCP should ask about safety, if the older adult feels safe driving alone, and if they feel safe driving with grandchildren or children in the car.

Although HCPs do not always feel comfortable discussing the idea of retiring from driving, there are times it is necessary to have the conversation. Approaching the subject of driving includes providing a supportive and comfortable environment, conversing directly with the patient, and not focusing on the patient's family or friends. In fact, when having the conversation, it is best to ask everyone in the room to leave but the patient. Reassure the patient the goal is to keep them mobile and safe within their environment [14]. Help them to take time to understand the goals of the driving-related appointments and let them know what a comprehensive driving evaluation entails and why it is needed. The HCP should be concerned about how the older adult health conditions may be affecting their driving. Starting the conversation by acknowledging the older adult's feelings and the driving concerns is recommended. If a family member is present, ask them if they would choose to let the patient in question drive them somewhere. If the answer is no, recommend further testing.

Screening

Screening is a brief method of identifying those at risk. It can be performed by the HCP in a formal manner during an appointment. There are also self-screenings the older adult or family member can access online at home. If there is a deficit noted by the older adult or family, a screening should be performed by the HCP during an appointment dedicated to this function. Screening for driving impairments should be done by the HCP after an illness, injury, or progressive changes in health.

The HCP plays a key role in assessing the individual to determine the potential cause of the driving impairment and ability. During the driving concern appointment with the HCP, a complete health history and physical examination should be done. The pathology of the impairment will help to determine whether the driving suspension is permanent or transient. If the HCP establishes there is a treatable cause that would benefit from rehabilitation, the patient may safely regain driving privileges in the future.

Health concerns like osteoarthritis, fractures, eye illness or injury, medication reactions, polypharmacy, recent surgeries, acute injuries, and recent illness all can lead to a temporary inability to drive, and may require driver rehabilitation and retesting instead of permanent license revocation. However, if there is a more severe pathology (amputation, low vision, severe progressive chronic illness, immobility, or cognitive decline) with a poor prognosis, the driving cessation can be permanent.

For HCPs, there are screenings that can be used for older adults during a dedicated appointment. The Mini Mental Status Examination is a commonly performed 30 question screening tool often administered to check for cognitive

Table 1	
Screening for Elder Driving Assessment	
Older adult driving screening assessment components	
Health history	Review of past medical, surgical, family, social, cultural histories
	Review current problem list
	In the social/lifestyle history note use of caffeine, nicotine, alcohol, or recreational drug use
Medication review	Review of all prescription medications including routine and as needed (prn)
	Over-the-counter medications, including liquids, rubs, lotions, etc
	Vitamins, minerals, herbs
	Home remedies
Physical examination	Comprehensive physical examination, including an eye examination
Mental status examination	Mini Mental Status Examination
	Trail Making (originated in the army in the 1940s) Consists of randomly placed numbered circles; older adult makes a trail by connecting the circles in numerical order and alternating letters and numbers
Common driving self-assessment products	
Fitness to Drive	Developed by University of Florida
	Available free online
	Web-based tool for caregivers and/or family members of older adult and HCP to identify at-risk older drivers
	http://fitnesstodrive.phhp.ufl.edu/us/
Drivers 65 Plus: Check Your Performance by AAA	Booklet with a self-assessment of driving
	Available free online
	http://seniordriving.aaa.com/wp-content/uploads/2016/08/Driver652.pdf

impairment [15]. Studies have shown that although having a patient copy intersecting pentagons is associated with a decline in driving skills, the rest of the Mini Mental Status Examination is not indicative of the ability to drive [16,17]. Table 1 lists some of the more commonly used screening tools.

It is the responsibility of the HCP to screen for risk and to examine the patient for an underlying curable cause; it is not the responsibility of the HCP to permanently remove an older adult driver's license. There are processes within each state where the HCP or the family can request a driving test through the Department of Motor Vehicles or Secretary of State, where driver's licenses are issued. In addition, a more comprehensive driving evaluation needs to be performed if driver safety is questioned.

Box 2: What is involved in a comprehensive driving assessment? [1,14]

Evaluator: OT-DRSs

Knowledgeable about progressive medical conditions, functional status and life changes that can affect driving

Components

- Clinical assessment
  - Includes a review of personal medical history, vision test, motor function, and cognitive assessment
  - Conducted by OT-DRSs
- Road test
  - Observance of traffic rules
    - Consistent use of strategies to compensate for impairments
  - Conducted by OT-DRSs or driving skills evaluator
- Oral feedback/written report
  - Results from the OT-DRS
    - May include treatment and intervention recommendations
    - Will indicate if older adult approved to drive, any modifications needed, any rehabilitation needed, or recommend cessation of driving

Cost

- $400+ for a full assessment [1].
- $100+ an hour for rehabilitation if needed [1]

Where to find a clinical driving assessment

Contact the American Occupational Therapy Association at https://myaota.aota.org/driver_search/index.aspx/index.aspx

From AAA. Senior Driving. 2020. Available at: https://seniordriving.aaa.com/ Accessed August 2, 2020; and Pomidor A, ed. Clinician's Guide to Assessing and Counseling Older Drivers, 4th edition. New York: The American Geriatrics Society; 2019.

Comprehensive driving evaluation assessment

A professional comprehensive driving assessment is a very thorough evaluation based on the older adult need and condition and usually consists of health history, review of systems, driving history, physical examination, and a clinical assessment of functional abilities, reflexes, and cognition. In addition, the comprehensive driving evaluation includes on-road testing with summary and recommendations, and a mobility plan. Although the HCP is able to screen for physical and mental problems that can cause driving impairments,

Table 2
Community resources

National Association of Area Agencies on Aging	Multiple resources available for older drivers Contact https://www.n4a.org/
DRS	OT-DRS or other health professional who will conduct a driving evaluation for a charge; works with older adult drivers who are in need of rehabilitation to resume driving
Department of Veterans Affairs	Driving rehabilitation program Information can be found at https://www.va.gov/VHAPUBLICAtIONs/ViewPublication.asp?pub_ID=5621
Department of Motor Vehicles or Secretary of State office	State agencies that will test older adult drivers with a request from an HCP or family member; may or may not be anonymous Search for your state agency
AAA (American Automobile Association)	Driver education refresher courses including update on the road rules and driving practice Many resources at https://seniordriving.aaa.com/
AARP (American Association of Retired People)	Driver Safety Programs Driver education refresher courses Many driving resources https://www.aarp.org/auto/driver-safety/
Car Fit Program	Through AAA, AARP and American Occupational Therapy Association sponsored community event that helps drivers adjust the fit of their car for safety Information at https://www.car-fit.org/
Alzheimer's Association Chapter	During mild dementia, a person can still drive but knowing their condition is progressive, hints are presented to know when it is time to abstain from driving https://www.alz.org/help-support/caregiving/safety/dementia-driving
Easter Seals Transportation along with the National Aging and Disability Transportation Center	Helps individuals find reasonable transportation https://www.easterseals.com/our-programs/transportation.html

in most US states the legal responsibility of retiring or removing driving privileges lies within the Department of Motor Vehicles or Secretary of State and is based on recommendations that result from the professional comprehensive driving evaluation performed by a health professional specializing in driving rehabilitation.

If the initial HCP screening shows there are concerns about the older adult driving safely, the next step would be a referral to an occupational therapist–driving rehabilitation specialist (OT-DRS) to complete the comprehensive driving evaluation. With specialized training in evaluating driving ability, these specialists evaluate, make plans, and will try to keep the patient mobile. Based on the evaluation results, if the patient is deemed not fit to drive, everyone needs to understand the older adult may be angry, hurt, and feel defeated. The components of a comprehensive driving evaluation are listed in Box 2.

RESOURCES FOR PROVIDERS TO OFFER FOR RETIRING DRIVERS

After the comprehensive driving assessment, the older adult will return to the HCP, who needs to allow the older adult who is a new nondriver time to process negative or hurt feelings. In addition, reassurance and support are needed for the older adult and family to plan for mobility resources. The older adult may need help creating a mobility plan if they have not yet started. It is crucial to ensure new older adult nondrivers have a plan for getting the important needs they are used to obtaining independently. Just as the teenager experiences a great rush of independence with the initiation of driving, the older adult frequently experiences grief at the loss of independence with the loss of driving privileges. It is important to approach this transition in life with dignity while preparing them to maintain a healthy lifestyle and socialization. At this point, the HCP can supply the older adult and family with resources needed to live a nondriving life.

Table 3
Transportation resources

Family and friends	Arrange rides; offer to bring supplies in; errands
Lyft or Uber	Ride services available for a fee
Taxi	Ride services available for a fee
Bus, subway, trains	Public transit, fee for service
Local senior citizen centers	Often have vans that offer ride share to older adult
Veterans groups; military lodges	If have military service record, may assist with transportation, especially to VA health care appointments
Religious or faith-based organizations	If a member of a certain organization, they may have volunteers that can provide rides or pick up to attend services/events
Door through Door services	Agencies provide drivers and escorts for help getting in and out of buildings; getting in and out of vans and cars for transport
Other organizations	May assist with transportation

There are many community resources available to assist with driving impairment which the HCP can provide. These resources are presented in Table 2 and are helpful in assessing the situation and providing for alternative transportation. Every practice with older adult should have a list of typical resources in a community or a handout that includes the following information with the local phone numbers.

Alternative transportation

Because the older adult will be retiring their driving privilege, it is best to provide them resources for transportation. Some resources are included in Table 3. Keep in mind that not every locale has public transportation or safe walkways. Not every retiring driver has family or friends available to drive them either.

Nutrition and Obtaining Food

The ability to drive affords one the freedom to purchase food whenever and at any time they want. Not driving means they may be at risk for running out of food and household supplies. Include menus and phone numbers for local delivery sources to maintain proper nutrition, hydration, and hygiene. Table 4 lists possible resources to present to patients and families to help them meet their nutritional needs if they are not driving.

Socialization

Keep in mind that no longer driving can be the equivalent of a teenager being grounded; they are at the mercy of someone else to let them visit others. People who are accustomed to an active social life will be at risk for isolation and depression. Encourage the retired driver to engage in social activities and know that providing rides to the local senior center, friend's homes and arranging rides will help. There are many ways to maintain socialization of a non-driving older adult including (keeping in mind that during the coronavirus

Table 4
Nutrition and supply services

Grocery delivery/Curbside pick-up	Many grocery stores offer call in or order and online grocery service with curbside pickup or delivery to home
Restaurant/pizza delivery	Many restaurants offer delivery
Door Dash or other meal delivery https://www.doordash.com/en-US	Door Dash is a company available in some locales with home delivery from various take out restaurants
Amazon or other mail delivery food delivery https://www.amazon.com/	Amazon offers online ordering with home delivery of groceries and supplies
Meals on Wheels https://www.mealsonwheelsamerica.org/	Local programs offering low-cost meals delivered to homes of older adult who meet the criteria
Have friends or family take the older adult to stores and restaurants or their homes for socialization (after the coronavirus disease 2019 pandemic)	Take them out to get supplies and enjoy their company!

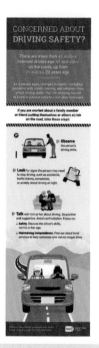

Fig. 1. Infographic. The US Department of Health and Human Services. National Institute on Aging website. Concerned about Driving Safety? [8].

disease 2019 restrictions, some of these opportunities may not be allowable or doable in some states or communities):

- Arranging a friend to pick the older adult up or come visit
- Making sure you are taking them out
- Stop by for a real visit and not for a task-oriented trip
- Phone calls, letters, emails, texting, and internet calls

SUMMARY

Mr P's children dealt with his declining health and unsafe driving by taking his keys. Mr R dealt with his wife's increased confusion and unsafe driving by not letting her drive alone. Mrs G's son dealt with gas/brake pedal issues and weakness by allowing her to continue to drive. All 3 of these people were at risk, and each one would have benefitted from having a plan in place to prepare for retirement from driving. The US Department of Health and Human Service's National Institute on Aging has produced an infographic [8] (Fig. 1) that can aid friends and families who are concerned about an older adult's ability to continue driving or prepare for retirement from driving.

Retirement from driving is a normal life stage and is associated with feelings of loss of freedom, independence, and self-reliance. Older adults who retire from driving without a plan are at risk for isolation, and depression leading to morbidity and possible mortality. If there is no plan for mobility, retiring driver patients are at risk for malnutrition and not getting the essentials they would normally go out and get themselves. It is best practice to begin driving retirement conversations early so patients are not surprised by the suggestion. As HCPs, we need to make this a normal element in life.

Disclosure

The author has no commercial or financial conflicts of interest and no funding sources.

References

[1] AAA. Senior Driving. 2020. Available at: https://seniordriving.aaa.com/. Accessed August 2, 2020.

[2] Federal Highway Administration, Department of Transportation (US). Highway Statistics 2017. Washington (DC): FHWA; 2018. Available at: https://www.fhwa.dot.gov/policy-information/statistics/2017/. Accessed 02 August 2020.

[3] Hedges & Company, 2020; Hudson, OH. Available at: https://hedgescompany.com/blog/2018/10/number-of-licensed-drivers-usa/. Accessed August 4, 2020.

[4] Mizenko AJ, Tefft BC, Arnold LS, et al. November). Older American drivers and traffic safety culture: a long road study. Washington, DC: AAA Foundation for Traffic Safety; 2014. Available at: https://aaafoundation.org/wp-content/uploads/2017/12/OlderAmericanDriversTrafficSafetyReport.pdf.

[5] Reisman A. surrendering the keys: a doctor tries to get an impaired elderly patient to stop driving. Health Aff (Millwood) 2011;30(2):356–9.

[6] Cicchino JB. Why have fatality rates among older drivers declined? The relative contributions of changes in survivability and crash involvement. Accid Anal Prev 2015;83:67–73.

[7] The Hartford. Your road ahead: a guide to comprehensive driving evaluations. 2012. Available at: https://s0.hfdstatic.com/sites/the_hartford/files/your-road-ahead-2012.pdf. Accessed August 2, 2020.

[8] Infographic US. Department of Health and Human Services. National Institute on Aging website. Concerned about Driving Safety?. Available at: https://www.nia.nih.gov/health/infographics/concerned-about-driving-safety. Accessed September 1, 2020.

[9] Betz ME, Scott K, Jones J, et al. Are you still driving?" Metasynthesis of patient preferences for communication with health care providers. Traffic Inj Prev 2016;17(4):367–73.

[10] Betz ME, Villavicencio L, Kandasamy D, et al. Physician and family discussions about driving safety: findings from the LongROAD study. J Am Board Fam Med 2019;32(4): 607–13.

[11] Huseth-Zosel AL, Sanders G, O'Connor M. Predictors of health care provider anticipatory guidance provision for older drivers. Traffic Inj Prev 2016;17(8):815–20.

[12] Harmon AC, Babulal G, Vivoda JM, et al. Planning for a nondriving future: behaviors and beliefs among middle-aged and older drivers. Geriatrics (Basel) 2018;3(2):19.

[13] Babulal GM, Vivoda J, Harmon A, et al. Older adults' expectations about mortality, driving life and years left without driving. J Gerontol Soc Work 2019;62(7):794–811.

[14] Pomidor A, editor. Clinician's guide to assessing and counseling older drivers. 4th edition. New York: The American Geriatrics Society; 2019.

[15] Pangman VC, Sloan J, Guse L. An examination of psychometric properties of the mini-mental status examination and the standardized mini-mental status examination: implications for clinical practice. Appl Nurs Res 2000;13(4):209–13.

[16] Barco P. Functional assessment of the older driver. Washington University Medical School; 2020 David B. Carr , MD.

[17] Health in Aging Foundation. HealthinAging.org. Top tips for Discussing when it's time to stop Driving. 2019. Available at: https://www.healthinaging.org/tools-and-tips/top-tips-discussing-when-its-time-stop-driving. Accessed August 2, 2020.

Vaccination Update for Nurse Practitioners Caring for Adults

Patrick C. Crane, DNP, RN, AGPCNP-BC

Michigan State University, College of Nursing, 1355 Bogue Street, Room A272, Life Sciences Building, East Lansing, MI 48824, USA

Keywords

- Vaccination • Immunization • Adult • Primary care • Disease prevention
- Wellness

Key points

- Vaccinations go through extensive safety research before being approved by the US Food and Drug Administration and the Centers for Disease Control and Prevention.
- Vaccinations are recommended across the lifespan to protect the population of the United States from serious disease.
- Vaccinations that are needed in adulthood are based on age, lifestyle, existing chronic conditions, and which vaccinations were received in childhood.
- The therapeutic relationship developed with patients in primary care is the best way for nurse practitioners to educate older adults on the importance of receiving timely vaccinations.

V accination has been an integral component to health promotion and prevention since the discovery of the smallpox vaccine in 1798 [1]. Throughout the history of vaccination and in contemporary time, much attention has been given to the importance of vaccination in population health owing to a vocal antivaccine movement, the spread of misinformation regarding the safety of vaccines, and growing numbers of preventable communicable diseases in the United States [2]. Moreover, there is currently a global effort to develop a vaccine for the prevention of the severe acute respiratory syndrome novel coronavirus 2, which has placed special attention on the role of vaccination in public health [3]. The necessity for primary care providers (PCP) to have a comprehensive understanding of vaccinations cannot be

E-mail address: cranepat@msu.edu

https://doi.org/10.1016/j.yfpn.2021.02.001

overstated. Partnering with patients to ensure they have access to accurate information and timely immunization is critical for health promotion and risk reduction.

The aim of this article is to provide PCP caring for adults a brief overview of crucial information needed to care for patients. This overview is not intended to be comprehensive, but rather to serve as a refresher for those who care for adults and older adults as a part of their patient panel. Vaccine basics such as administration schedules and clinical implications for patient vaccination such as holding patient conversations regarding vaccination and vaccination myths are discussed.

The most important way to set a foundation for this article is introducing the reader to the common definitions used when discussing vaccinations. The definitions are in Table 1.

PHYSIOLOGY OF VACCINE
Understanding the role of the immune system in the induction of immunity from vaccines is important to review. Immunization, in general, primarily takes advantage of the adaptive immune system of the human body. This is beneficial to preventing infectious diseases as the adaptive immune system can develop a memory against certain pathogens [5].

Among the most critical biological components that produce an active immunity within the human body is that of humoral immunity. The physiology of humoral immunity uses B cells to produce antibodies, which are often referred to as immunoglobins (Ig). B cells are produced in bone marrow and migrate to lymph nodes. The binding of an antigen with a B cell induces the B cell to differentiate into a plasma cell, producing antibodies at a rate of around 2000 antibody molecules per second [6,7]. Some B cells can also require activation via T-helper cells. When needed, T-helper cells can induce additional

Table 1 Vaccine definitions	
Word	Definition and example
Live-attenuated vaccine	A vaccine that uses a weakened form of virus that causes disease
	Examples include the varicella, measles, mumps, rubella [4]
Inactivated vaccine	A vaccine that uses a virus that is, no longer able to reproduce
	Examples include hepatitis A and injectable influenza vaccines [4]
Subunit, recombinant, polysaccharide, and conjugate vaccine	A vaccine that uses a specific piece of a disease-causing germ such as a protein, capsid or sugar, to provide protection against certain diseases
	Examples include hepatitis B and shingles vaccines [4]
Toxoid vaccine	A vaccine that uses a toxin made by a disease-causing organism that has been treated to no longer create a toxic effect to provide immunity through antibody formation [4]

activation of B cells to produce a stronger immune response [5]. Producing memory cells for a long-term and strong immune response is the overall goal of immunization.

On initial presentation of an antigen, and over the course of several days, antigen-specific IgM antibodies are produced via cloning of plasma cells [5]. The presence of IgM antibodies also signifies the acute phase of the infection. Over several months, IgG antibodies are produced and are generally better at neutralizing antigens opsonization for phagocytosis and activation of the complement system. Upon subsequent exposures to the antigen, IgG will mediate a quicker and heightened secondary immune response [5].

Cell-mediated immunity serves as the other component of active immunity. The major function of cell-mediated immunity is to protect the body from intracellular pathogens such as viruses. The major components of cell-mediated immunity are CD4 and CD8 T cells. Cell-mediated immunity does not involve the secretion of antibodies but, upon exposure, uses major histocompatibility complexes to identify intracellular pathogens. T cells become activated when pathogens using major histocompatibility complexes are presented on the surface of a cell that also contains self-antigens. After exposure to a pathogen, cell-mediated immunity helps to suppress viral replication until primary T-cell responses are mounted or to alert and activate B cells for an immune response against the pathogen [8]. Amanna and Slifka [8] note that many of the first successful vaccines used this technique for developing human immunity to specific pathogens.

VACCINATION SCHEDULE FOR ADULTS
The US Centers for Disease Control and Prevention (CDC) is currently the leading authority on adult vaccination in the United States. The CDC publishes recommended vaccine schedules to ensure that patients receive needed protection from infectious disease in a timely and evidence-based fashion. The CDC publishes this schedule yearly at https://www.cdc.gov/vaccines/schedules/hcp/imz/adult.html [9]. Fig. 1 presents the most current adult vaccine schedule at the time of publication. In addition to the recommended schedule of immunization, the CDC publishes regular updates and guidance to both patients and providers regarding vaccines and immunizations. The CDC web site further provides print outs, reference materials, and resources that may be useful to providers in their practice.

Hepatitis A
Hepatitis A (HAV) is a communicable viral infection that causes inflammation of the liver and is transmitted through the fecal–oral route. HAV accounts for nearly one-third of all viral hepatitis cases in developed countries [10]. HAV infection in the United States had decreased by more than 95% from 1995 until 2011; however, since 2016 the incidence has sharply increased [11]. More than 75% of adults remain asymptomatic while they are infected [10]. This statistic

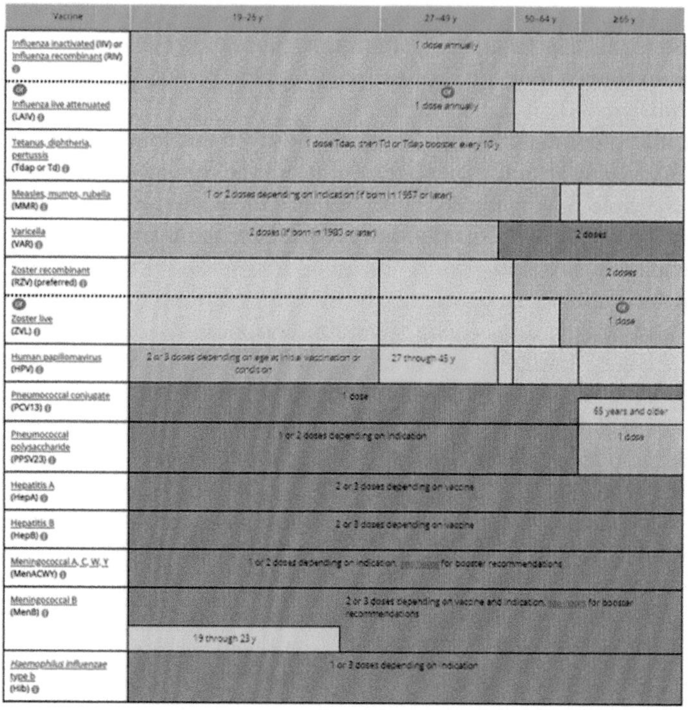

Fig. 1. CDC Adult immunization schedule. Yellow: Recommend vaccination for adults who meet age requirement, lack documentation of vaccination, or lack evidence of past infection Purple: Recommend vaccination for adults with an additional risk factor or another indication Blue: Recommend vaccination based on shared clinical decision-making. Gray: No recommendation or N/A. (Centers for Disease Control and Prevention. *Recommended adult immunization schedule for ages 19 years or older, United States.* Available at https://www.cdc.gov/vaccines/schedules/hcp/imz/adult.html#note-hpv.)

underscores why providers should be familiar with HAV vaccination guidelines and encourage immunization to their patients.

According to the CDC, the people most at risk for HAV infection are those who travel internationally, men who have sex with men, people who use illegal drugs, those who have occupational risk for exposure, people who anticipate personal contact with an international adoptee, and people experiencing homelessness [11]. Incarcerated individuals are additionally at an increased risk for viral hepatitis infection [10].

The HAV vaccine (HepA) has been part of the routine childhood immunization schedule since 1994 [12]. Because this vaccine was introduced to the schedule in relatively recent times, providers are likely to encounter large numbers of adults who have not received a HepA vaccine as a part of their routine care. For those individuals who have not been infected with HAV and who have not been vaccinated, the CDC recommends 2 doses of the Havrix vaccine 6 to 12 months apart, or 2 doses of the Vaqta vaccine 6 to 18 months apart [13]. Both Vaqta and Havrix are inactivated, single-antigen vaccines. In addition to the single antigen vaccine, there is also an approved bivalent HAV and hepatitis B vaccine (Twinrix) that is given in 3 doses. Twinrix is given at 0-, 1-, and 6-month intervals to complete the series. Twinrix contains hepatitis A antigen in a lower dose than in the noncombination vaccines and may be a viable option if the patient requires protection from both hepatitis A and hepatitis B [13]. Providers should be familiar with the incidence and prevalence of hepatitis A in their community and encourage those adults in endemic areas to become vaccinated.

Important contraindications to consider
- Havrix and Vaqta are both contraindicated in individuals with latex and neomycin allergies.
- Latex is a component of the vaccine packaging.
- Neomycin is used in the manufacturing process of the HepA vaccine.

Hepatitis B
Hepatitis B (HBV), like HAV, is a viral, communicable infection that causes inflammation in the liver [14]. Unlike HAV however, HBV can become a chronic, lifelong infection in some individuals [14]. Particularly concerning is that HBV infection was reported as an underlying or contributing cause of death in more than 1600 individuals in 2018 [15]. This finding is mostly due to the HBV being a major risk factor for developing liver cirrhosis or hepatocarcinoma [16]. The virus is often transmitted from mother to child during birth or through contact with blood or other body fluids of an infected individual [17]. Currently, it is estimated that approximately 850,000 individuals are chronically infected with HBV; the CDC estimates there are approximately 20,900 acute infections of HBV in the United States [18]. Despite these statistics, only about 25% of adults older than19 years of age are vaccinated against HBV in the United States [19]. Providers must be familiar with the significant underimmunization of adults in their country and implement clinic reminders to discuss immunization against HBV during routine office visits. Unimmunized adults at risk for contracting HBV are people who use injection drugs, individuals who have sex with partners infected with HBV, men who have sex with men, people who cohabitate with an HBV-positive individual, health care and public safety workers who may be exposed to blood, and hemodialysis patients [15].

The CDC currently recommends vaccination for those adults who are not at risk for HBV but want protection, and for those who are at risk for contracting HBV [9]. There are currently 2- and 3-dose single-antigen, recombinant vaccines on the market. The 2-dose series (Heplisav-B), should be given at least 4 weeks apart [9]. The 3-dose series (Engerix-B or Recombivax HB), should be given at 0, 1, and 6 months [9]. There is also a licensed 3-dose HAV–HBV vaccine (Twinrix) that may be an option for those who require protection from HAV and HBV. Clinicians should refer to Table 2 for dosing recommendations.

Table 2
Recommended doses of currently licensed formulations of hepatitis B vaccine for adults

| Age group | Single-antigen vaccine | | | | | | Combination vaccine | |
| | Recombivax HB | | Engerix-B | | Heplisav-B | | Twinrix[a] | |
	Dose (µg)[b]	Vol (mL)	Dose (µg)[b]	Vol (mL)	Dose (µg)[b]	Vol (mL)	Dose (µg)[b]	Vol (mL)
Adults (≥18 y)					20	0.5	20[a]	1
Adults (≥20 y)	10	1	20	1	20	0.5	20[a]	1
Hemodialysis patients and other immunocompromised persons <20 y[c]	5	0.5	10	0.5	20	0.5	NA	NA
≥20 y	40[d]	1	40[e]	2.0	20	0.5	NA	NA

[a]Combined hepatitis A and hepatitis B vaccine. This vaccine is recommended for people aged ≥18 y who are at increased risk for both hepatitis B virus and hepatitis A virus infections.

[b]Recombinant hepatitis B surface antigen protein dose.

[c]Higher doses might be more immunogenic, but no specific recommendations have been made.

[d]Dialysis formulation administered on a 3-dose schedule at 0, 1, and 6 mo.

[e]Two 1.0-mL doses administered at one site, on a 4-dose schedule at 0, 1, 2, and 6 mo.

Adapted from the 2020 CDC table *What are the Recommended Doses of hepatitis B Vaccines?* Retrieved from https://www.cdc.gov/hepatitis/hbv/hbvfaq.htm.

Important contraindications to consider
- Caution should be used in individuals with allergies to yeast and latex because these components are used in the manufacturing and packaging of these products [20,21].
- Heplisav-B is not recommended for use in pregnant women because there is a lack of safety data in this population [9].

Human papillomavirus
Human papillomavirus (HPV) is the most common communicable, sexually transmitted infection in the United States. The CDC estimates that nearly 79 million Americans are infected with HPV [22]. HPV has been identified as a cause of cancers of the genitals, anus, and oropharynx [22]. HPV strains 16 and 18 are responsible for nearly 70% of all cervical cancer cases [23]. In 2006, the US Food and Drug Administration approved GARDASIL, the first vaccine for 4 types of HPV (16, 18, 6, and 11). In 2009, CERVARIX, a bivalent vaccine, was approved to protect against HPV 16 and 18 [23,24]. In 2014 a 9-valent vaccine, Gardasil 9, was approved by the US Food and Drug Administration and is currently the only licensed HPV vaccine available in the United States [25]. In addition to protection from the high-risk cancer-causing strains of HPV, both the quadrivalent and 9-valent vaccines offer some additional protection from low-risk, wart-causing HPV strains [25,26]. All currently approved HPV vaccines use virus-like particles formed by the surface components of HPV without containing any DNA from the virus [26,27].

HPV vaccination rates remain disparate among men and women. In females 19 to 26 years of age, 48.5% reported receipt of at least 1 HPV vaccine dose, whereas only 13.5% males of the same age reported receiving at least 1 dose of an HPV vaccine [19]. Because of the relatively low rates of immunization, PCPs should address the recommendation for HPV vaccination in both females and males aged 15 to 45 years of age. However, dosing recommendations for the administration of HPV vaccine differ among age groups. Adding further confusion is that the number of doses varies based on the age at initial vaccination [9]. For anyone beginning the series before their 15th birthday, the CDC recommends 2 doses of the HPV vaccine at least 6 months apart. Those beginning the series from their 15 to 45 years of age require a 3-dose series at 0, 2, and 6 months [9]. Table 3 provides an overview of HPV vaccination based on age at first dose.

There are many misconceptions that a PCP may encounter regarding the HPV vaccine [29]. Among these are that the HPV vaccine can cause infertility or HPV infection [30]. As the CDC notes, the HPV vaccine is a recombinant vaccine and incapable of creating an active infection [30]. Additionally, multiple studies have found no link between infertility caused by the HPV vaccine [30,31]. For parents who worry that HPV vaccination may lead to sexual promiscuity, evidence has also refuted this claim [32].

Important contraindications to consider
  • Gardasil 9 is contraindicated in individuals who are allergic to yeast, which is used in the manufacturing process [28].

Influenza

Influenza ("the flu") is a contagious respiratory disease that is, spread through droplets when people cough, sneeze, or talk. Additionally, it can be spread by encountering infected surfaces or objects, and then touching one's mouth or nose [33]. On average, influenza causes symptoms in about 8% of the US population each year [34]. Although older adults tend to have a lower incidence of influenza than younger individuals, their rate of hospitalization and mortality from influenza is much higher than those who are less than 65 years old [35]. Although older adults tend to carry the burden of morbidity and mortality related to influenza, younger adults with health conditions such as pregnancy, diabetes, and heart and lung disease, are also at risk for complications from influenza [36]. Despite these figures, the CDC estimates that only 45.3% of adults in the United States were vaccinated during the 2018/2019 flu season [37].

The CDC recommends annual influenza vaccination for all people greater than 6 months of age with any influenza vaccine appropriate for the patient's age and health status [9,38]. Furthermore, the timing of influenza vaccine administration should occur early in the fall, before the virus begins spreading in communities [38].

The influenza vaccine is available in multiple forms and formulations. Those that are most administered in clinical settings are the inactivated influenza vaccine, quadrivalent recombinant influenza vaccine, and the quadrivalent live

Table 3
Recommended schedule of HPV vaccine by population

Recommended number of doses	Recommended dosing schedule[c]	Population
2	0, 6–12 mo[a]	Persons initiating vaccination at ages 9–14 y, except immunocompromised persons
3	0, 1–2, 6 mo[b]	Persons initiating vaccination at ages 15–26 y Immunocompromised persons initiating vaccination at ages 9–26 y Adults initiating vaccination at ages 27–45 y

[a]In a 2-dose schedule of HPV vaccine, the minimum interval is 5 mo between the first and second doses.
[b]In a 3-dose schedule of HPV vaccine, the minimum intervals are 4 wk between the first and second doses, 12 wk between the second and third dose, and 5 mo between the first and third dose.
[c]All doses are 0.5 mL [28].
  Adapted from the 2020 CDC table *Vaccine Administration.* Available at https://www.cdc.gov/vaccines/vpd/hpv/hcp/administration.html.

attenuated influenza vaccine. The inactivated influenza vaccine and quadrivalent recombinant influenza vaccine vaccines are administered intramuscularly, whereas the quadrivalent live attenuated influenza vaccine is dosed via an intranasal spray. The inactivated influenza vaccine has been approved for those older than 6 months of age, and the quadrivalent recombinant influenza vaccine is licensed only for those individuals who are at least 18 years old. PCPs should also be aware the quadrivalent live attenuated influenza vaccine has only been approved for those 2 to 49 years of age. Finally, for those patients 65 years old or greater, a high-dose, inactivated trivalent vaccine is available. This vaccine contains 4 times the antigens of the standard dose vaccine and has been shown to generate a stronger immune response in older adults [39].

Important contraindications to consider
- Live attenuated influenza vaccine should not be used in immunocompromised individuals, people with anatomic or function asplenia, those with cochlear implants, patients with cerebrospinal fluid–oropharyngeal communication, those whose close contacts or caregivers are immunocompromised, pregnant individuals, or those treated with antiviral medications for influenza within the previous 48 hours [9].
- If patient is severely allergic to eggs, influenza vaccination should only be administered in a setting where providers can recognize and manage allergic reactions [9].
- Unless vaccination benefits outweigh the risk, people with a history of Guillain–Barré syndrome within 6 weeks of a previous vaccine should not be vaccinated [9].

Measles, mumps, and rubella
Measles virus is an exceptional respiratory disease caused by the genus *Morbillivirus* and spread through direct respiration or aerosol [40]. Although measles is often regarded as a childhood disease, nearly 1 in 5 unvaccinated people in the United States who contract measles become hospitalized [41]. Owing to a strong vaccination program, measles virus was declared eliminated in 2000 in the United States [42]. However, owing to the spread of measles virus in communities of unvaccinated individuals, and outbreaks in countries where Americans often travel, there has been a recent increase in measles virus infection in the United States [43].

Mumps is a contagious viral illness that is caused by a Paramyxovirus and is spread by respiratory droplets [44]. Although, like measles virus, often considered a childhood illness, some outbreaks have been noted among patients in their 20s and 30s [44]. Adults with mumps tend to develop more severe illness and are at an increased risk for complications associated with the virus [45]. Complications include deafness, orchitis in males, and oophoritis in females [45]. Despite a highly effective vaccine, multiple outbreaks have been noted in the United States [45].

Rubella virus, also known as German measles, is a togavirus and is transmitted through the inhalation of infected droplets [44]. The virus can cause a viral syndrome, including arthritis in 70% of females; however, 25% to 50% of all cases are asymptomatic [44,46]. However, the main concern regarding rubella virus infection is that it has a tendency to produce teratogenic effects, especially if the mother is infected in the first trimester [44,46]. Congenital rubella syndrome often leads to deafness, heart defects, intellectual disabilities, low birth weight, and liver and spleen damage [46]. Furthermore, congenital rubella syndrome increases the risk of miscarriage or stillbirth [46]. Rubella virus was declared eliminated in the United States in 2014; however, isolated cases continue to be recorded in the United States, mostly among unvaccinated people arriving from other countries [44].

In 1998, Wakefield, and colleagues [47] published an article in the February issue of *The Lancet* that contributed significantly to the myth that the measles, mumps, and rubella (MMR) vaccine is linked to autism [48]. This article, despite being retracted by *The Lancet* in 2010, continues to generate misinformation about the fraudulent link between receiving the MMR vaccine and the development of autism [48]. Multiple studies have been published and have consistently found no such link [48–50]. Among so much misinformation perpetuated by 1 article, it is imperative that PCP are confident, accurate, and upfront with patients when confronted with questions regarding the safety of the MMR vaccine.

Currently, vaccines against measles, mumps, and rubella are combined into a combined vaccine (MMR II) in the United States. This is a live vaccine and thus special caution should be taken for those individuals with immunocompromising conditions as described elsewhere in this article. There is an additional live vaccine that includes varicella (ProQuad); however, this vaccine has not approved for use in adults in the United States.

The CDC recommends 1 dose of the MMR in adults without evidence of immunity to MMR [9]. Evidence of immunity includes documentation of MMR vaccination or laboratory evidence of immunity [9]. There are several situations where the number of doses varies based on the health status of the individual. Table 4 should be referenced for clinician guidance regarding these cases. The CDC further describes health care workers as a special population. Those health care personnel born before 1957 without evidence of immunity to MMR are recommended to receive a 2-dose series, 4 weeks apart for measles or mumps or 1 dose for rubella [9]. Those born in 1957 or later should receive a 2-dose series at least 4 weeks apart for measles or mumps or at least 1 dose of MMR for rubella [9].

Important contraindications to consider

- Contraindicated in persons with HIV infection with a CD4 count of less than 200 cells/μL [9].
- Contraindicated in persons with severe immunocompromising conditions [51].
- Do not administer in persons with active, untreated tuberculosis [51].
- Do not administer to persons with an active febrile illness with a fever greater than 101.3°F [51].

Table 4
MMR special situation dosing

Recommended number of doses	Recommended dosing schedule[a]	Situation
1	N/A	Pregnancy without evidence of immunity to rubella. Nonpregnant women of childbearing age without evidence of immunity to rubella. Postsecondary students, international travelers, and household/personal contacts or immunocompromised persons if previously received 1 dose of MMR.
2	0, 4 wk	HIV infection with a CD4 count of ≥200 cells/µL for ≥6 mo and no evidence of immunity to rubella. Postsecondary students, international travelers, and household/personal contacts or immunocompromised persons without evidence of immunity to measles, mumps, or rubella.

[a]All doses are 0.5 mL administered subcutaneously [51].
  Adapted from: Centers for Disease Control and Prevention. Recommended Adult Immunization Schedule for Ages 19 years or older, United States, 2020. Available at https://www.cdc.gov/vaccines/schedules/hcp/imz/adult.html.

- Do not administer to individuals who are pregnant or who are planning on becoming pregnant within the first month [51].

Meningococcal

Meningitis is an inflammation of the meninges and caused by multiple organisms including viruses and bacteria [10]. Among the most common causative bacteria are *Streptococcus pneumoniae*, group B *Streptococcus*, *Neisseria meningitidis*, *Hemophilus influenzae*, and *Listeria monocytogenes* [52,53]. *N meningitidis* is a meningococcus that is categorized into 13 serogroups where groups A, B, C W135, and Y are involved in most cases of invasive disease, with Y being the most predominant subgroup in the United States [54]. *N meningitidis* is spread via respiratory sections through coughing, kissing, or living in close contact for prolonged periods of time [52]. Licensed meningitis vaccines in the United States focus on these 5 common serogroups. Other vaccines such as the pneumococcal vaccine and *H influenzae* type B vaccine help to protect individuals from other bacteria that are common causes of meningitis [52].

Although cases of meningococcal disease in the United States are decreasing, adolescents and young adults aged 16 to 23 years have the highest rates of disease [55]. The CDC also notes that up to 15 in 100 people who become infected with meningococcal disease will die and 1 in 5 survivors will experience a long-term disability such as deafness, brain damage, nervous system disorders, or loss of limbs [55]. For this reason, PCPs should identify those at risk and ensure that they receive immunization to protect against these adverse outcomes.

Adult risk factors for contracting meningitis include gatherings of large groups, such as living on college campuses, immunocompromising conditions or medications, traveling to sub-Saharan Africa, or being employed in a setting where one is routinely exposed to meningitis-causing bacteria [52]. PCP should identify risk factors in their adult patient population to determine the need for immunization.

PCP caring for adult patients should recognize that the CDC recommends all preteens receive a meningitis A-C-W-Y (MenACWY) vaccine at ages 11 to 12 years old [56]. This vaccination is followed by a booster at 16 years of age. Providers who care for adolescents should ensure that their 16-year-old patients have received the complete series.

Two licensed MenACWY vaccines are available in the United States: meningococcal (groups A, C, Y, and W-135) polysaccharide diphtheria (Menactra) and meningococcal (groups A, C, Y, and W-135) oligosaccharide diphtheria (Menveo) [57]. Both vaccines are approved for persons aged 2 to 55 years of age. It is important to note that neither of these vaccines provide immunity to the meningococcal group B (MenB) virus.

There are 2 approved MenB vaccines licensed in the United States: MenB-FHbp (Trumenba) and MenB-4C (Bexsero). Both vaccines have been approved for persons 10 to 25 years of age [58,59]. Adolescents 16 to 23 years of age who are not at increased risk for meningococcal disease, should engage in shared decision-making with their PCP to determine the need for immunization. For those wishing to become vaccinated, the CDC recommends a 2-dose series of MenB-4C at least 1 month apart, or 2 doses of MenB-FHbp at 0 and 6 months [9]. If the second dose of MenB-Fhbp was given less than 6 months after the initial dose, a third dose should be given 4 months after dose 2 [9]. However, be aware that MenB-4C and MenB-FHbp cannot be used interchangeably, so the same product needs to be used for the entire series [9].

Some special considerations for which adults should be vaccinated against meningitis B exist. Functional and anatomically asplenic patients, individuals with sickle cell disease, those with persistent complement component deficiency, or those prescribed a complement inhibitor should receive a 2-dose series of MenB-4C at least 1 month apart, or a 3-dose series of MenB-FHbp at 0, 1 to 2, and 6 months [9]. If dose 2 of MenB-FHbp was administered at least 6 months after dose 1, the third dose is not required [9]. Finally, people such as microbiologists who work with *Neisseria meningitidis* are recommended to receive the same series of vaccines for those who are asplenic (citation 6) [9].

Important contraindications to consider
- MenACWY is contraindicated in persons with severe allergy to MenACWY vaccine components, including diphtheria toxoid [60].
- Providers should delay administering MenACWY in anyone with moderate or severe acute illness [60].

- Delay MenB until after pregnancy unless the patient is at risk and the benefits outweigh the risks [9].

Pneumococcal

Pneumonia is an infection of the lower respiratory tract and caused by a variety of organisms including *Streptococcus pneumonia, Mycoplasma pneumoniae, H influenzae*, and *Chlamydophila pneumoniae*, as well as multiple respiratory viruses [10]. Older adults tend to be the most vulnerable to community-acquired pneumonia in the United States owing to comorbidities and declining immune function [10]. Despite high mortality from pneumonia, the CDC estimates that only 60% to 70% of adults greater than 65 year old and 18% to 24% of younger adults at risk for pneumonia are vaccinated against it [19]. Common risk factors for the development of pneumonia include adults 65 years or older, people with chronic medical conditions, individuals who smoke cigarettes, those who are addicted to alcohol, and people with HIV infection [10,61].

In 2019, the Advisory Committee on Immunization Practices changed their recommendations regarding routine vaccination for adults 65 years old and older [62]. Previously, it was recommended that all adults 65 years old and older receive a series of 2 pneumonia vaccines; a 13-valent pneumococcal conjugate vaccine (PCV13) sold under the trade name Prevnar 13, followed by a 23-valent pneumococcal polysaccharide vaccine (PPSV23) sold under the trade name Pneumovax 23 [62]. The Advisory Committee on Immunization Practices now recommends against the routine use of the PCV13 vaccine in older adults and instead recommends that the same population receive 1 dose of PPSV23 [62]. However, the Advisory Committee on Immunization Practices encourages shared clinical decision-making with patients to determine if PCV13 is right for a certain individual [62]. The CDC notes that if both PCV13 and PPSV23 are administered, the PCP should administer PCV13 first, followed by PPSV23 1 year later [9].

PCPs face further decision-making because there are several instances where pneumococcal vaccination should occur before age 65. Individuals aged 19 to 64 years with chronic heart disease, lung disease, liver disease, diabetes, alcoholism, or who are cigarette smoking should receive 1 dose of PPSV23 [9]. Individuals with immunocompromising conditions or anatomic/functional asplenia should receive 1 dose of PCV13, followed by 1 dose of PPSV23 at least 8 weeks apart. Another dose of PPSV23 should be given 5 years after the previous PPSV23, then a final dose of PPSV23 after reaching age 65 at least 5 years after the previous PPSV23 [9]. Finally, individuals with cerebrospinal fluid leak or cochlear implant should receive 1 dose of PCV13 followed by 1 dose of PPSV23 at least 8 weeks later. A final dose of PPSV23 should be given at age 65 at least 5 years after the previous dose of PPSV23 [9].

Important contraindications to consider

- Do not administer if the patient has had a severe allergic reaction to any diphtheria toxoid-containing vaccine as this is a component of PPSV23 [63].

Tetanus, diphtheria, and pertussis

Tetanus disease is a bacterial infection caused by *Clostridium tetani* [64]. The disease is often fatal, and its symptoms include muscle rigidity, muscular spasms, and the classic symptom of lockjaw [64]. Since the 1940s, when the first vaccine was introduced, cases of tetanus dramatically decreased in the United States [64]. In 2009, only 18 cases of tetanus were identified in the United States and of those, most had never been vaccinated or had not received a booster dose [64].

Diphtheria is a bacterial disease caused by strains of *Corynebacterium diphtheriae* [65]. Diphtheria can involve almost any mucous membrane, involve the respiratory tract or skin, and is usually characterized by sore throat, nasal discharge, hoarseness, fever, and malaise [44]. Although the nasal infection chiefly results in nasal discharge, laryngeal diphtheria can result in airway and bronchial obstruction [44,65]. Diphtheria can also lead to serious complications, including myocarditis, heart failure, neuritis, slurred speech, difficulty swallowing, and death [44,65]. Diphtheria remains relatively rare in the United States with only 5 cases being reported since 2000 [65]. However, diphtheria remains active in other parts of the world [65]. Most providers may never see a case of diphtheria owing to its relative rarity in the United States; however, those caring for adult populations, particularly immigrants, should be aware of the immunization status of their patients and encourage immunization when needed.

Pertussis, also known as whooping cough, is a respiratory tract infection caused by the *Bordetella pertussis* bacteria and transmitted through respiratory droplets [44,66]. Pertussis, like tetanus and diphtheria is a toxin-mediated disease [64–66]. The disease typically follows a series of stages, where in 1 to 6 weeks, the paroxysmal stage is reached [66]. In this stage, the hallmark bursts or rapid coughing, followed by a high-pitched, deep inspiration (whoop) is noted [44]. Frequent coughing can persist for up 10 weeks after infection [66]. Adult deaths from pertussis are rare; however, adolescents and adults can experience complications including urinary incontinence, pneumonia, rib fractures, and sleep disruption [66].

Effective vaccines against tetanus (1924), diphtheria (1920s), and pertussis (1914) were developed as toxoid vaccines in the early part of the twentieth century [64–66]. In the United States today, vaccines against tetanus, diphtheria, and pertussis are available in one vaccine (Tdap) sold under the trade names Boostrix and Adacel [64]. Adacel is approved for persons 10 to 64 years of age, and Boostrix is approved for those individuals 10 years old and older [64]. Additionally, 2 combined tetanus and diphtheria toxoid (Td) vaccines are available in the United States for adult use; a generic and Tenivac [64]. Both preparations are approved for people 7 years of age and older [67,68].

The CDC recommends routine vaccination for those who have not previously received primary vaccination against tetanus, diphtheria, or pertussis to receive one dose of Tdap, followed by 1 dose of Td or Tdap 4 weeks after the first dose, then 1 dose of Td or Tdap 6 to 12 months after the previous dose

[9]. If patients did not receive Tdap at age 11, it is recommended to administer 1 dose of Tdap, then boost with Tdap or Td every 10 years [9]. Additionally, a tetanus toxoid-containing vaccine should be used as a component of wound management if more than 5 years have passed since the last Td or Tdap dose [69]. Finally, the CDC recommends 1 dose of Tdap during each pregnancy, with administration at 27 to 36 gestational weeks being preferred [9].

Important contraindications to consider
- This is a moderate to severe acute illness.
- Tdap is contraindicated in people with a history of encephalopathy without another identifiable cause occurring within 7 days of receiving a pertussis-containing vaccine [65].
- Precaution should be used in patient with a history of Guillain-Barré syndrome within 6 weeks of receiving a tetanus toxoid-containing vaccine and a progressive neurologic disorder [65].

Varicella
Varicella zoster virus (VZV), or chickenpox is a highly contagious disease that often occurs in childhood [70]. Although only about 2% of all cases of VZV occur in those more than 20 years of age, this age group accounts for nearly one-half of all deaths from VZV [70]. Among the most serious and life-threatening complication of VZV infection is the development of pneumonia [71]. The varicella vaccine (VAR) was introduced in 1995 as a 1-dose vaccination, and in 2006, a second dose was recommended as part of the vaccination schedule [72]. Although the VAR has contributed to a dramatic decrease in VZV rates, there likely remains a small percentage of adults who do not have a known history of varicella disease or varicella vaccination [72]. PCPs need to inquire about known exposure to disease and vaccination status among their patients.

Currently, the only licensed single antigen VAR in the United States is approved for adult populations. This vaccine is sold under the trade name Virivax [73]. The CDC recommends a 2-dose series 4 to 8 weeks apart if an individual has not been immunized against varicella and has no evidence of immunity, and was born before 1980 [9]. If an individual has evidence of only receiving 1 dose of VAR, a second dose should be given at least 4 weeks after their first dose [9]. Patients who are health care workers should also follow these recommendations but should receive the vaccine even if they were born before 1980 and have no evidence of immunity [9].

PCP of individuals with HIV with a CD4 count of 200 cells/µL or greater can consider VAR administration, but the schedule should be modified to 2-dose series, 3 months apart [9].

Important contraindications to consider
- VAR is contraindicated during pregnancy [9].
- VAR is contraindicated in those with severe immunocompromising conditions [9].

- VAR is contraindicated in HIV infection with a CD4 count of less than 200 cells/µL [9].
- VAR is contraindicated in febrile illness and active infection, including untreated tuberculosis [74].
- VAR is contraindicated in patients allergic to neomycin and gelatin because they are components of the vaccine [74].
- Recommend against use of salicylates in people 12 to 17 years of age for 6 weeks after vaccination [74].
- Defer vaccination for at least 5 months after blood/plasma transfusions or the administration of immune globulins [74].

Herpes zoster

Herpes zoster (HZ), also known as shingles, is a skin eruption that is caused by reactivation of the VZV, which lies dormant in the dorsal root ganglia for years to decades after a primary infection with VZV [10]. HZ results in a painful or pruritic rash that typically occurs on the trunk, but can also involve the face or, in some cases, present without a rash [10]. HZ is quite common in the United States with approximately 1 million cases reported each year [75]. The CDC estimates that 1 out of 3 people will develop HZ in their lifetime [76]. The incidence of HZ increases as individuals age with an incidence 1 case per 100 persons over age 60 [76].

Serious complications can result from an HZ outbreak. About 10% of patients 60 to 69 years old will develop postherpetic neuralgia, a debilitating neuropathic pain that results from damage to the sensory nerves [77,78]. This complication occurs in 20% of those with HZ who are 80 years of age and older [77]. Additionally, adults with suppressed immune systems are more likely to be hospitalized as a result of HZ infection and, although rare, are more likely to die of the infection [76]. Further complications include vision loss as well as cranial and peripheral nerve palsies [76].

Two vaccines for HZ are currently licensed in the United States. The first, zoster live vaccine (ZVL, Zostavax) was first licensed in 2006 but will no longer be available for sale in the United States after July 1, 2020 [76,78]. In 2018, the Advisory Committee on Immunization Practices recommended use of the newer zoster vaccine recombinant, adjuvanted (RZV, Shingrix) in 2 doses beginning at age 50 [79].

The CDC currently recommends a 2-dose series of RZV 2 to 6 months apart with a minimum interval of 4 weeks from the first dose for patients 50 years or older. This is recommended even if patients have a previous history of ZVL vaccination [9]. However, RZV should not be administered sooner than 2 months after vaccination with ZVL [9].

The Advisory Committee on Immunization Practices reported that the RZV prevented HZ in approximately 97% of vaccinated individuals and prevent postherpetic neuralgia in 91% of the vaccinated population [79]. Because of the demonstrated efficacy of RZV, PCPs should encourage their patients who are 50 years or older to receive RZV even if they have previously been vaccinated with ZVL.

Important contraindications to consider
- There is no available safety data in regard to the RZV vaccine in pregnant and lactating women [79].
- Do not administer when a patient has a current HZ infection [79].

SPECIAL CONSIDERATIONS
Older adults
Older adults experience declining immune response and higher morbidity and mortality from infectious diseases such as influenza and pneumonia [35,80]. Older adults are also disproportionately affected by HZ [76]. Despite these facts, only 66.9% of older adults are vaccinated against pneumonia, 33.4% against HZ, and 70.4% against influenza [19]. The PCP must partner with patients and their caregivers to ensure that they receive recommended vaccines in a timely fashion.

Socioeconomic factors may play a role in patients' ability to receive required vaccines. Although some routine vaccines are covered by Medicare part B (influenza, pneumococcal, HepB) vaccines such as shingles and Tdap are only covered under a Medicare advantage (Medicare part D) plan [81,82]. This factor is particularly problematic because only about 31% of all Medicare beneficiaries are enrolled in an advantage plan [83]. Additionally, 14.6% of all older adults live below the poverty level [84], which may impair their ability to travel to clinics or pharmacies to receive annual wellness or immunization visits or to pay out of pocket for immunizations.

Other reasons that older adults do not become vaccinated are that they are unaware of their increased vulnerability, the do not feel urgency because their health care provider has not encouraged vaccination, they worry that vaccines might make them ill, or their PCP office does not stock vaccines and they were not referred to an office that does [85]. PCPs should provide an opportunity for patients to discuss their questions and rationale for their hesitancy in becoming vaccinated.

Lesbian, gay, bisexual, transgender, and queer persons
Little literature exists on specific immunization protocols for the lesbian, gay, bisexual, transgender, and queer (LGBTQ+) community. Specific immunizations that PCP should encourage among LGBTQ+ populations revolve around sexually transmitted infectious disease risks specific to this community. Specifically, PCP should ensure HPV, HepB, and HepA vaccination among their LGBTQ+ patients [86]. The US Department of Health and Human Services further recommends influenza vaccine for gay or bisexual men [87], but makes no specific recommendation for lesbian, transsexual, bisexual, or queer women. A PCP must be aware of their patient's sexual behaviors, sexual orientation, and gender identity to build trusting relationships and further ensure health promotion and disease prevention among this population. Additionally, PCPs should partner with scientists to better close the gap in the literature regarding immunization and the LGBTQ+ community.

Ethnic disparities

Racial and ethnic disparities have been described in the literature [88,89]. Adult vaccination, in general, was lower in Black, Hispanic, and Asian populations when compared with non-Hispanic Whites [88]. Factors that contribute to this disparity include attitudes toward vaccination and preventative care, differences in how ethnic minorities seek and accept vaccination, differences in the overall quality of care received, and differences in perceived vaccine safety [88]. Additionally, socioeconomic differences play a role in vaccination rates among minority populations, including higher rates of uninsured [90].

PCPs must ensure that they are playing an active role in decreasing disparities among non-White patients. Providers should, again, ensure that there are opportunities during a visit to discuss the need for vaccination. Additionally, allowing for discussions to assess and address misconceptions will likely be beneficial in patient's consent to receive scheduled vaccination. Furthermore, as with all patient populations, developing a trusting, 2-way relationship between the PCP and the patient is essential to help ensure better vaccine coverage.

IMPLICATIONS FOR CLINICAL PRACTICE

Talking with patients about vaccination

As discussed briefly elsewhere in this article, the publication of the Wakefiled and colleagues [47] has spurred unwarranted controversy regarding the safety of vaccines. Additional misconceptions to specific vaccines such as HPV have been addressed throughout this article as well. Now, more than ever, PCPs need to be prepared to address these misconceptions and educate their patients on the evidence supporting vaccine safety. In addition to addressing common misconceptions regarding vaccines, PCP will encounter numerous other questions or concerns from patients regarding vaccination.

Dudley and colleagues [91] provide an in-depth overview of how to discuss vaccines with patients. They recommend a 5-step strategy when working with patients who are hesitant to receive vaccines. These strategies are outlined in Table 5.

Misconceptions are not the only reason that patients choose not to become vaccinated. As discussed elsewhere in this article, socioeconomic factors also may play a role. During vaccine conversations with patients, the PCP should communicate low-cost or free vaccine clinics within the local area. Having print materials with dates, hours, and locations of such clinics may be useful in reinforcing the patient to visit.

Finally, the PCP should be persistent in their conversations with patients regarding vaccinations. Continually reinforcing the importance of vaccination along with addressing individual barriers with patients is likely to keep the issue top of mind for unvaccinated individuals.

Ensuring vaccination of patients in the clinical setting

It is recommended that PCP create a culture of immunization within their practice [92]. The National Vaccine Advisory Committee standards call on all

Table 5
Strategies for working with vaccine hesitant patients

Provide empathy and credibility	Be understanding, but do not affirm a myth or misperception when establishing empathy. Use motivational interviewing techniques.
Address the patient's specific concerns	Discuss what you have read and/or learned from the literature and other scientific sources.
Discuss the risks of disease	Share the severity and susceptibility to the disease that vaccines can protect against
Convey the effectiveness of the vaccine(s) you are recommending	Emphasize what can be done to protect against disease
	Pair discussions of disease risk with self-efficacy and a call to action. Assure the patient one of the best actions they can take to prevent communicable disease.
Personalize your recommendation	Offer that you strongly recommend the vaccination and that you would also do so to your friends and family. You may want to discuss if your family has received the vaccine you are recommending.

Adapted from Dudley MZ, Salmon DA, Halsey NA, et al. The Clinician's Vaccine Safety Resource Guide: Optimizing Prevention of Vaccine-Preventable Diseases Across the Lifespan. Springer; 2018 [91].

health care professionals to assess the immunization status of all patients at every clinical encounter, for PCPs to strongly recommend vaccines that the patient needs, to administer required vaccinations or refer patients to a vaccination provider, and finally to document the vaccines received by your patients [82].

Structural methods of better ensuring vaccination coverage in practices include implementing systems to incorporate vaccination assessment into routine clinical care, ensuring providers know how to access immunization information on their patients, have methods for ensuring professional competencies in immunizations, and developing referral relationships with providers for those clinics that do not offer vaccination [82]. PCP also need to ensure that they remain up to date and educate their patients on vaccine recommendations [82].

Coronavirus disease 2019

The recent severe acute respiratory syndrome novel coronavirus 2 pandemic has highlighted the important role vaccines play in the prevention of communicable diseases. A vaccine against coronavirus disease 2019 (COVID-19) has been identified as a "global imperative" and is likely a requirement for societies to return to normal in countries where the virus continues to thrive [93]. The US government has created a private–public partnership program titled Operation Warp Speed to mobilize resources to create and deliver 300 million doses of a COVID-19 vaccine by January 2021 [94]. As of September, 10 2020, 25 vaccines were in phase I trials, 14 in phase II, 9 in phase III, and 3 vaccines had been approved for early or limited use [95]. At the date of writing, only 1 (COVID-19) vaccine has been approved globally. On August 11, 2020, the Ministry of Health of the Russian Federation approved a COVID-19 vaccine (Sputnik V) [96]. However, concerns regarding the vaccine's safety and efficacy have been called into question owing to approval of the vaccine before the completion of phase II trials [97,98].

It is difficult to predict if, at the time of printing, an approved and licensed COVID-19 vaccine will be available in the United States. If researchers and manufactures prevail in this monumental task, it will likely appear on the adult vaccine schedule soon thereafter. PCPs will need to be informed of the indications, contraindications, and special considerations for adult populations when such a vaccine is approved. Undoubtedly, like with current vaccines, there will be many questions.

SUMMARY

Vaccination is a crucial component of health promotion and disease prevention. PCPs play a critical role to ensure that the population receives the recommended immunizations at the recommended time. Vaccines are licensed, phased out, and recommendations are changed frequently. For this reason, it is critical that the PCP remain up to date on current recommendations for vaccines. PCPs should also ensure that structures and processes are incorporated into their practices to optimize the number of patients who become immunized. Finally, skillful communication is needed to address patient's misconceptions, questions and concerns. Keeping these principles in mind, PCP can best continue their mission to provide high-quality primary care.

Disclosure

The author has nothing to disclose.

References

[1] Plotkin S. History of vaccination. Proc Natl Acad Sci U S A 2014;111(34):12283–7.
[2] Dubé E, Vivion M, MacDonald NE. Vaccine hesitancy, vaccine refusal and the anti-vaccine movement: influence, impact and implications. Expert Rev Vaccines 2015;14(1):99–117.
[3] McKeever A. Dozens of COVID-19 vaccines are in development. Here are the ones to follow. National Geographic. 2020. Available at: https://www.nationalgeographic.com/science/health-and-human-body/human-diseases/coronavirus-vaccine-tracker-how-they-work-latest-developments-cvd/. Accessed August 31, 2020.
[4] US Department of Health & Human Services. Vaccine types. 2020. Available at: Vaccines.gov; https://www.vaccines.gov/basics/types. Accessed September 11, 2020.
[5] Clem AS. Fundamentals of vaccine immunology. J Glob Infect Dis 2011;3(1):73–8.
[6] Sherwood L. Fundamentals of physiology: a human perspective. Belmont (CA): Brooks Cole; 2006.
[7] Goldsby RA, Kindt TJ, Osborne BA, et al. B-cell generation, activation, and differentiation. Immunology 2003;5:266–74.
[8] Amanna IJ, Slifka MK. Contributions of humoral and cellular immunity to vaccine-induced protection in humans. Virology 2011;411(2):206–15.

[9] Centers for Disease Control and Prevention. Recommended adult immunization schedule for ages 19 years or older, United States, 2020. 2020. Available at: CDC.gov; https://www.cdc.gov/vaccines/schedules/hcp/imz/adult.html. Accessed August 6, 2020.

[10] Buttaro TM, Trybulski J, Bailey PP, et al. Primary care: a collaborative approach. 4th edition. St Louis (MO): Elsevier; 2013.

[11] Centers for Disease Control and Prevention. Hepatitis A questions and answers for health professionals. 2020. Available at: CDC.gov; https://www.cdc.gov/hepatitis/HAV/HAV-faq.htm#A2. Accessed August 7, 2020.

[12] Roush SW, Baldy LM, Kirkconnell Hall MA, College of Physicians of Philadelphia. The history of vaccines: hepatitis A and hepatitis B. 2018. Historyofvaccines.org. Available at: https://www.historyofvaccines.org/content/articles/hepatitis-and-hepatitis-b. Accessed August 8, 2020.

[13] Centers for Disease Control and Prevention. Recommended Adult Immunization Schedule for ages 19 years or older, United States, 2020. 2020. Available at: CDC.gov; https://www.cdc.gov/vaccines/schedules/hcp/imz/adult-conditions.html#note-hepa. Accessed August 14, 2020.

[14] Centers for Disease Control and Prevention. Viral Hepatitis. 2020. Available at: CDC.gov; https://www.cdc.gov/hepatitis/hbv/bfaq.htm. Accessed August 14, 2020.

[15] Centers for Disease Control and Prevention. Hepatitis B questions and answers for health professionals. 2020. Available at: CDC.gov; https://www.cdc.gov/hepatitis/hbv/hbvfaq.htm. Accessed August 21, 2020.

[16] Hilleman MR. Critical overview and outlook: pathogenesis, prevention, and treatment of hepatitis and hepatocarcinoma caused by hepatitis B virus. Vaccine 2003;21(32): 4626–49.

[17] World Health Organization. Hepatitis B. 2020. Available at: WHO.int; https://www.who.int/news-room/fact-sheets/detail/hepatitis-b. Accessed July 27, 2020.

[18] Department of Health and Human Services. Hepatitis B Basic Information. 2020. Available at: HHS.gov; https://www.hhs.gov/hepatitis/learn-about-viral-hepatitis/hepatitis-b-basics/index.html. Accessed August 21, 2020.

[19] Centers for Disease Control and Prevention. Vaccination coverage among adults in the United States, National Health Interview Survey, 2016. 2018. Available at: CDC.gov; https://www.cdc.gov/vaccines/imz-managers/coverage/adultvaxview/pubs-resources/NHIS-2016.html. Accessed August 21, 2020.

[20] Engerix-B. Package insert. GlaxoSmithKline;1989.

[21] Recombivax HB. Package insert. Merck & Co., Inc.;2018.

[22] Centers for Disease Control and Prevention. Genital HPV Infection Fact Sheet. 2019. Available at: CDC.gov; https://www.cdc.gov/std/hpv/stdfact-hpv.htm. Accessed August 21, 2020.

[23] Villa LL. HPV prophylactic vaccination: the first years and what to expect from now. Cancer Lett 2011;305(2):106–12.

[24] The College of Physicians of Philadelphia. The history of vaccines: human papillomavirus infection. Historyofvaccines.org. 2018. Available at: https://www.historyofvaccines.org/content/articles/human-papillomavirus-infection. Accessed August 21, 2020.

[25] Centers for Disease Control and Prevention. Human Papillomavirus (HPV) vaccine: vaccine safety. 2020. Available at: CDC.gov; https://www.cdc.gov/vaccinesafety/vaccines/hpv-vaccine.html. Accessed August 21, 2020.

[26] National Cancer Institute. Human Papillomavirus (HPV) vaccines. 2019. Available at: Cancer.gov; https://www.cancer.gov/about-cancer/causes-prevention/risk/infectious-agents/hpv-vaccine-fact-sheet#how-do-hpv-vaccines-work. Accessed August 21, 2020.

[27] Hildesheim A, Herrero R, Wacholder S, et al. Effect of human papillomavirus 16/18 L1 viruslike particle vaccine among young women with preexisting infection: a randomized trial. JAMA 2007;298(7):743–53.

[28] Gardasil 9 package insert. Merck & Co., Inc.; 2020.

[29] Bednarczyk RA. Addressing HPV vaccine myths: practical information for healthcare providers. Hum Vaccin Immunother 2019;15(7-8):1628-38.

[30] Centers for Disease Control and Prevention. Human papillomavirus: HPV vaccination is safe and effective. 2019. Available at: CDC.gov; https://www.cdc.gov/hpv/parents/vaccine-safety.html. Accessed September 11, 2020.

[31] Schmuhl NB, Mooney KE, Zhang X, et al. No association between HPV vaccination and infertility in U.S. females 18-33 years old. Vaccine 2020;38(24):4038-43.

[32] Coles VA, Patel AS, Allen FL, et al. The association of human papillomavirus vaccination with sexual behaviours and human papillomavirus knowledge: a systematic review. Int J STD AIDS 2015;26(11):777-88.

[33] Centers for Disease Control and Prevention. Key facts about influenza (flu). 2019. Available at: CDC.gov; https://www.cdc.gov/flu/about/keyfacts.htm. Accessed August 6, 2020.

[34] Tokars JI, Olsen SJ, Reed C. Seasonal incidence of symptomatic influenza in the United States. Clin Infect Dis 2018;66(10):1511-8.

[35] Wilhelm M. Influenza in older patients: a call to action and recent updates for vaccinations. Am J Manag Care 2018;24(2 Suppl):S15-24.

[36] Centers for Disease Control and Prevention. People at high risk for flu complications. 2020. Available at: CDC.gov; https://www.cdc.gov/flu/highrisk/index.htm. Accessed August 6, 2020.

[37] Centers for Disease Control and Prevention. Flu vaccination coverage, United States, 2018-2019 influenza Season. 2019. Available at: CDC.gov; https://www.cdc.gov/flu/fluvax-view/coverage-1819estimates.htm. Accessed August 6, 2020.

[38] Centers for Disease Control and Prevention. Who should and who should not get a flu vaccine. 2019. Available at: CDC.gov; https://www.cdc.gov/flu/prevent/whoshouldvax.htm#anchor_1555704832. Accessed August 7, 2020.

[39] DiazGranados CA, Dunning AJ, Kimmel M, et al. Efficacy of high-dose versus standard-dose influenza vaccine in older adults. N Engl J Med 2014;371(7):635-45.

[40] Naim HY. Measles virus. Hum Vaccin Immunother 2015;11(1):21-6.

[41] Centers for Disease Control and Prevention. Complications of measles. 2019. Available at: CDC.gov; https://www.cdc.gov/measles/symptoms/complications.html. Accessed August 30, 2020.

[42] Centers for Disease Control and Prevention. Measles history. 2018. Available at: CDC.gov; https://www.cdc.gov/measles/about/history.html. Accessed August 30, 2020.

[43] Centers for Disease Control and Prevention. Questions about measles. 2019. Available at: CDC.gov; https://www.cdc.gov/measles/about/faqs.html. Accessed August 30, 2020.

[44] Papadakis MA, McPhee SJ, Rabow MW, editors. Current medical diagnosis & treatment 2019. New York: McGraw-Hill; 2019.

[45] Clemmons N, Hickman C, Lee A, et al. Chapter 9: mumps. In: Manual for the surveillance of vaccine-preventable diseases. Atlanta (GA): Centers for Disease Control and Prevention; 1996. Available at: https://www.cdc.gov/vaccines/pubs/surv-manual/chpt09-mumps.html. Accessed August 30, 2020.

[46] Centers for Disease Control and Prevention. Pregnancy and rubella. 2017. Available at: CDC.gov; https://www.cdc.gov/rubella/pregnancy.html. Accessed August 30, 2020.

[47] Wakefield AJ, Murch SH, Anthony A, et al. Ileal-lymphoid-nodular hyperplasia, non-specific colitis, and pervasive developmental disorder in children. Lancet 1998;351(9103):637-41 [retracted in: Lancet. 2010;375(9713):445].

[48] Flaherty DK. The vaccine-autism connection: a public health crisis caused by unethical medical practices and fraudulent science. Ann Pharmacother 2011;45(10):1302-4.

[49] Di Pietrantonj C, Rivetti A, Marchione P, et al. Vaccines for measles, mumps, rubella, and varicella in children. Cochrane Database Syst Rev 2020;(4):CD004407.

[50] Institute of Medicine (US), Immunization Safety Review Committee. In: Stratton K, Gable A, Shetty P, et al, editors. Immunization safety review: measles-mumps-rubella vaccine and autism. Washington, DC: National Academies Press (US); 2001.

[51] M-M-R II. Package insert. Merck & Co., Inc.; 2020.

[52] Centers for Disease Control and Prevention. Meningitis. 2019. Available at: CDC.gov; https://www.cdc.gov/meningitis/bacterial.html. Accessed September 9, 2020.

[53] Centers for Disease Control and Prevention. Haemophilus influenzae type b. In: Atkinson W, Wolfe S, Hamborsky J, et al, editors. Epidemiology and prevention of vaccine-preventable diseases. 13th edition. Washington, DC: Public Health Foundation; 2009. p. 119–34. Available at: https://www.cdc.gov/vaccines/pubs/pinkbook/hib.html. Accessed September 11, 2020.

[54] McGill F, Heyderman RS, Panagiotou S, et al. Acute bacterial meningitis in adults. Lancet 2016;388(10063):3036–47.

[55] Centers for Disease Control and Prevention. Meningococcal disease: clinical information. 2019. Available at: CDC.gov; https://www.cdc.gov/meningococcal/clinical-info.html. Accessed September 9, 2020.

[56] Centers for Disease Control and Prevention. Meningococcal disease: meningococcal vaccination. 2020. Available at: CDC.gov; https://www.cdc.gov/meningococcal/vaccine-info.html. Accessed September 10, 2020.

[57] Centers for Disease Control and Prevention. Vaccines and preventable diseases: meningococcal vaccination. 2019. Available at: CDC.gov; https://www.cdc.gov/vaccines/vpd/mening/index.html. Accessed September 10, 2020.

[58] Trumenba. Package insert. Pfizer; 2018.

[59] Bexsero. Package insert. GlaxoSmithKline; 201x.

[60] Centers for Disease Control and Prevention. Meningococcal disease. In: Atkinson W, Wolfe S, Hamborsky J, et al, editors. Epidemiology and prevention of vaccine-preventable diseases. 13th edition. Washington, DC: Public Health Foundation; 2009. p. 231–46. Available at: https://www.cdc.gov/vaccines/pubs/pinkbook/mening.html. Accessed September 11, 2020.

[61] Centers for Disease Control and Prevention. Pneumonia can be prevented – Vaccines can help. 2019. Available at: CDC.gov; https://www.cdc.gov/pneumonia/prevention.html#:~:text=There%20are%20two%20vaccines%20that,pneumococcal%20disease%3A%20PCV13%20and%20PPSV23.&text=CDC%20recommends%20all%20adults%2065,get%20a%20shot%20of%20PPSV23. Accessed September 10, 2020.

[62] Matanock A, Lee G, Gierke R, et al. Use of 13-valent pneumococcal conjugate vaccine and 23-valent pneumococcal polysaccharide vaccine among adults aged ≥65 years: updated recommendations of the Advisory Committee on Immunization Practices. MMWR Morb Mortal Wkly Rep 2019;68(46):1069–75 [published correction appears in MMWR Morb Mortal Wkly Rep 2020;68(5152):1195].

[63] Prevnar 13. Package insert. Pfizer; 2017.

[64] Centers for Disease Control and Prevention. Tetanus. In: Atkinson W, Wolfe S, Hamborsky J, et al, editors. Epidemiology and prevention of vaccine-preventable diseases. 13th edition. Washington, DC: Public Health Foundation; 2009. p. 341–52. Available at: https://www.cdc.gov/vaccines/pubs/pinkbook/downloads/tetanus.pdf. Accessed September 11, 2020.

[65] Centers for Disease Control and Prevention. Diphtheria. In: Atkinson W, Wolfe S, Hamborsky J, et al, editors. Epidemiology and prevention of vaccine-preventable diseases. 13th edition. Washington, DC: Public Health Foundation; 2009. p. 107–18. Available at: https://www.cdc.gov/vaccines/pubs/pinkbook/dip.html. Accessed September 11, 2020.

[66] Centers for Disease Control and Prevention. Pertussis. In: Atkinson W, Wolfe S, Hamborsky J, et al, editors. Epidemiology and prevention of vaccine-preventable diseases. 13th edition. Washington, DC: Public Health Foundation; 2009. Available at: https://www.cdc.gov/vaccines/pubs/pinkbook/pert.html. Accessed September 11, 2020.

[67] Tetanus and diphtheria toxoids absorbed. Package insert. MassBiologics; 2018.

[68] Tenivac. Package insert. Sanofi Pasteur Limited; 2019.

[69] Liang JL, Tiwari T, Moro P, et al. Prevention of pertussis, tetanus, and diphtheria with vaccines in the United States: recommendations of the Advisory Committee on Immunization Practices (ACIP). MMWR Recomm Rep 2018;67(2):1.

[70] Preblud SR. Varicella: complications and costs. Pediatrics 1986;78(4 Pt 2):728–35.

[71] Guess HA, Broughton DD, Melton LJ 3rd, et al. Population-based studies of varicella complications. Pediatrics 1986;78(4 Pt 2):723–7.

[72] Bialek SR, Perella D, Zhang J, et al. Impact of a routine two-dose varicella vaccination program on varicella epidemiology. Pediatrics 2013;132(5):e1134–40.

[73] Centers for Disease Control and Prevention. Vaccine safety: chickenpox (Varicella) vaccines. 2020. Available at: CDC.gov; https://www.cdc.gov/vaccinesafety/vaccines/varicella-vaccine.html. Accessed September 10, 2020.

[74] Virivax. Package insert. Merck & Co., Inc.; 1995.

[75] Insinga RP, Itzler RF, Pellissier JM, et al. The incidence of herpes zoster in a United States administrative database. J Gen Intern Med 2005;20(8):748–53.

[76] Centers for Disease Control and Prevention. Shingles (herpes zoster). 2020. Available at: CDC.gov; https://www.cdc.gov/shingles/hcp/clinical-overview.html. Accessed September 11, 2020.

[77] Yawn BP, Saddier P, Wollan PC, et al. A population-based study of the incidence and complication rates of herpes zoster before zoster vaccine introduction. Mayo Clin Proc 2007;82(11):1341–9 [published correction appears in Mayo Clin Proc 2008;83(2):255].

[78] Sampathkumar P, Drage LA, Martin DP. Herpes zoster (shingles) and postherpetic neuralgia. Mayo Clin Proc 2009;84(3):274–80.

[79] Dooling KL, Guo A, Patel M, et al. Recommendations of the Advisory Committee on Immunization Practices for Use of Herpes Zoster Vaccines. MMWR Morb Mortal Wkly Rep 2018;67(3):103–8.

[80] Andrew MK, Bowles SK, Pawelec G, et al. Influenza vaccination in older adults: recent innovations and practical applications. Drugs Aging 2019;36(1):29–37.

[81] Centers for Disease Control and Prevention. Medicare part D vaccines. 2019. Available at: CMS.gov; https://www.cms.gov/Outreach-and-Education/Medicare-Learning-Network-MLN/MLNProducts/Downloads/Vaccines-Part-D-Factsheet-ICN908764.pdf. Accessed September 12, 2020.

[82] National Vaccine Advisory Committee. Recommendations from the National Vaccine Advisory committee: standards for adult immunization practice. Public Health Rep 2014;129(2):115–23.

[83] Jacobson G, Neuman T, Freed M, et al. What percent of new Medicare beneficiaries are enrolling in Medicare Advantage?. 2019. Available at: KFF.org; https://www.kff.org/medicare/issue-brief/what-percent-of-new-medicare-beneficiaries-are-enrolling-in-medicare-advantage/. Accessed September 12, 2020.

[84] DeNavas-Walt C, Proctor BD. Income and poverty in the United States: 2013. Washington, DC: US Government Printing Office; 2014.

[85] American College of Physicians. Aging and immunity: the important role of vaccines. American College of Physicians. Available at: https://www.acponline.org/system/files/documents/clinical_information/resources/adult_immunization/aging_and_immunity_guide.pdf. Accessed September 12, 2020.

[86] Mathews J. LGBTQ Pharmacy Guide. St. John Fisher College. 2016. Available at: https://fisherpub.sjfc.edu/cgi/viewcontent.cgi?article=1081&context=pharmacy_facpub. Accessed September 12, 2020.

[87] US Department of Health and Human Services. Vaccines for gay or bisexual men. Vaccines.gov. Available at: https://www.vaccines.gov/who_and_when/gay_or_bisexual_men. Accessed September 12, 2020.

[88] Lu PJ, O'Halloran A, Williams WW, et al. Racial and ethnic disparities in vaccination coverage among adult populations in the U.S. Vaccine 2015;33(Suppl 4):D83–91.

[89] Walker AT, Smith PJ, Kolasa M, et al. Reduction of racial/ethnic disparities in vaccination coverage, 1995-2011. MMWR Suppl 2014;63(1):7–12.

[90] DeNavas-Walt C, Proctor BD, Lee CH. Income, poverty, and health insurance coverage in the United States (2005). Washington, DC: US Government Printing Office; 2006.

[91] Dudley MZ, Salmon DA, Halsey NA, et al. The clinician's vaccine safety resource guide: optimizing prevention of vaccine-preventable diseases across the lifespan. New York: Springer; 2018.

[92] Centers for Disease Control and Prevention. Immunization strategies for healthcare practices and providers. In: Atkinson W, Wolfe S, Hamborsky J, et al, editors. Epidemiology and prevention of vaccine-preventable diseases. 13th edition. Washington, DC: Public Health Foundation; 2009. p. 33–46. Available at: https://www.cdc.gov/vaccines/pubs/pinkbook/strat.html. Accessed September 11, 2020.

[93] Graham BS. Rapid COVID-19 vaccine development. Science 2020;368(6494):945–6.

[94] US Department of Health and Human Services. Fact sheet: explaining operation warp speed. 2020. Available at: HHS.Gov; https://www.hhs.gov/about/news/2020/06/16/fact-sheet-explaining-operation-warp-speed.html. Accessed September 12, 2020.

[95] Corum J, Grady D, Sui-Lee W, et al. Coronavirus vaccine tracker. New York Times 2020. Available at: https://www.nytimes.com/interactive/2020/science/coronavirus-vaccine-tracker.html. Accessed September 11, 2020.

[96] Craven J. Covid-19 vaccine tracker. Regulatory Affairs Professional Society. 2020. Available at: https://www.raps.org/news-and-articles/news-articles/2020/3/covid-19-vaccine-tracker. Accessed September 12, 2020.

[97] Zimmer C. 'This is all beyond stupid.' Experts worry about Russia's rushed vaccine. New York Times 2020. Available at: https://www.nytimes.com/2020/08/11/health/russia-covid-19-vaccine-safety.html. Accessed September 12, 2020.

[98] Lovelace B Jr. Scientists worry whether Russia's "Sputnik V" coronavirus vaccine is safe and effective. CNBC 2020. Available at: https://www.cnbc.com/2020/08/11/scientists-worry-whether-russias-sputnik-v-coronavirus-vaccine-is-safe-and-effective.html. Accessed September 12, 2020.

Obstructive Sleep Apnea in Older Adults
Diagnosis and Management

Nina Ganesh Nandish, AGPCNP-BC*, Nilan Nandish

Adult and Gerontological Primary Care Medicine, 14555 Levan Road, Suite 308, Livonia, MI 48154, USA

Keywords

- Obstructive sleep apnea in older adults • Hypopnea • Sleep disorders
- Excessive daytime sleepiness • Hypersomnia • Hypersomnolence • C-PAP
- COVID-19

Key points

- Sleep is an important factor in every unique individual's overall health, well-being, and quality of life.
- A common sleep disorder, obstructive sleep apnea, is underdiagnosed, inaccurately diagnosed, and inappropriately treated in older adults who experience both normal changes of aging and the impact of chronic comorbid conditions on airways leading to obstruction.
- Nurse practitioners and other health care professionals need to question older adults about their sleep habits, sleep hygiene, functional and cognitive status, and history of falls and accidents and document the information.
- Older adults, 70 and older, with obstructive sleep apnea have an increased mortality and a shorter survival time.

INTRODUCTION

"Man is the only mammal that willingly delays sleep" [1]. Sleep is often misunderstood, in part because all human beings have unique individual sleep requirements depending on genetics, physiologic factors, sleep experience, age, gender, and lifestyle, to name a few. Some people like to sleep a lot; some vigorously fight sleeping, and others wish there were more hours in the day so they could accomplish tasks and still get an adequate amount of sleep. Where do you fall? In order to learn about sleep alterations or deviations, it is important to review some basic information about sleep.

*Corresponding author. E-mail address: nnandish22@gmail.com

https://doi.org/10.1016/j.yfpn.2021.01.002
2589-420X/21/© 2021 Elsevier Inc. All rights reserved.

There are many misconceptions about the purpose of sleep and how much one needs. Sleep is not about the brain shutting down; there are important pathophysiologic mechanisms taking place while one is sleeping. Restoration, consolidating and storing memories, muscle growth, rejuvenation, organ system fortification, tissue repair, and hormone synthesis represent some of the brain activity that normally occurs during sleep. Restful sleep is critical in order to maintain good mental, emotional, physical, and spiritual health as well as cognitive alertness. It is a myth that one can *catch up* from sleep deprivation over a weekend. Another myth is that as one gets older, they require less sleep; this statement is not true! Too much sleep can have a negative impact on one's metabolism and can increase the risk of back pain, cardiovascular (CV) disease, headache, and obesity [2].

Thus, what are the current recommendations for the optimal amount of sleep time adults need? The Centers for Disease Control and Prevention (CDC) support the National Sleep Foundation sleep time duration recommendations [3]. The recommended hours of sleep for adults are shown in Table 1. As always, it is imperative to approach each adult patient as a unique individual. Given the patient's family history, lifestyle, abilities, functional status, and presence of any chronic conditions, the nurse practitioner (NP) will want to determine what the best duration (amount) of evidence-based (EB) sleep is for each individual person.

It is important to keep in mind that the fastest aging population globally is the oldest old, which is ≥85 years. This age cohort has different sleep patterns and sufficiency needs but will not be addressed in this article.

Despite recommendations, short sleep duration (<7 hours of sleep in 24 hours) persists in the United States and is reported by approximately 35% of all adults (2017). The CDC called insufficient sleep *a public health epidemic* in 2008; sleep satisfaction among adults has decreased since that statement [4]. In 2017, Abraham and colleagues reported poor satisfaction with sleep and increased heath care–seeking behaviors related to lack of sleep in older adults (OA) [5].

With aging, there are sleep architectural (functional patterns) changes. Normal aging changes related to sleep include the following:

- Changes in the circadian cycle/rhythm (the body's internal clock) leading to earlier sleep onset [6]
- Increase in the time it takes to fall asleep (sleep latency)
  - Going to bed when tired is more beneficial than tossing and turning while trying to fall asleep

Table 1
Recommended hours of sleep

Age group/range	Hours of sleep
Young adult: 18–25 y	7–9
Adult: 26–64 y	7–9
Older adult: 65 y and older	7–8

- Decreased ability to maintain sleep leads to less total sleep time
  - Increased number of awakenings and earlier morning wake signal
  - Prolonged nocturnal awakenings, including increased nocturia (sleep fragmentation)
- Shortened nocturnal sleep duration
- Decreased deep sleep (slow wave sleep or rapid eye movement [REM] sleep), which is the most refreshing stage of sleep
  - OAs spend most of their time in lighter versus deeper sleep stages [3,7]

Incorporating beneficial sleep habits or sleep hygiene into one's life is how one can gain maximum benefit from time spent sleeping (sleep duration). Good sleep hygiene consists of the following:

- Getting up and going to bed at the same time every day, including weekends
  - Maintaining a consistent pattern/schedule
- Ensuring the room where sleep occurs is dark, relaxing, and quiet, with a comfortable (cooler) temperature
  - Noise can be eliminated with the use of a fan, white noise machine, earplugs, headphones, and so forth
- Removing stimulating smells from the room and adding soothing smells if they assist in falling asleep
- Not eating or snacking in bed
- Avoiding large, spicy meals and alcohol at least 3 hours before bedtime
- Avoiding nicotine and caffeine; both are stimulants that interfere with sleep
- Toileting just before bedtime
- Avoiding interruptions from lighting
  - Black out curtains and sleep masks can both block light and prevent it from interfering with sleep
- Removing electronic devices from the room
  - Light from devices can suppress natural production of melatonin (a hormone that promotes sleep)
  - Devices include television, computer, smart phone, tablet, blue screens, and so forth
  - Disconnect at least 30 minutes before intended bedtime
- Winding down for 30 minutes before sleep allows the brain to relax
  - Low-impact stretching
  - Listen to soothing music
  - Quiet reading
  - Relaxation exercises
  - Meditation, guided imagery
  - Mindfulness (being in the moment)
- Using the bed for sleep and intimate relationships only
- Using a quality mattress, pillow, and bedding (need to be replaced on a regular basis)
- Maintaining a nutritional diet
- Engaging in physical activity throughout the day
- Napping for short, versus long, periods of time
- Creating a pre–bedtime routine or schedule and following it every day [1,8].

Educating patients about sleep hygiene and having conversations about how many daily hours of sleep is optimal will provide the needed facts the OA needs to think about restful sleep in order to maintain maximum mind-body-spirit health.

There are more than 80 different sleep disorders, and the prevalence increases with age [9]. The American Sleep Association [10] determined that 50 to 70 million adults in the United States experience sleep disorders. These disorders are not related to normal aging but rather to medications, chronic conditions, either physical or mental, lifestyle, and other factors the NP will need to discover through therapeutic listening and appropriate age-based questioning. Many OA report dissatisfaction with their quality or daily amount of sleep and *do not feel well rested in the morning.* This question is the most important question that the NP needs to ask the OA patient during an office visit regarding sleep.

Sleep disorders are conditions that impact normal patterns of sleep. Not getting enough sleep can be caused by underlying conditions, such as CV disease, type 2 diabetes, and obesity (CDC, 2020). Some of the more prevalent adult sleep disorders are found in Table 2.

The second most common sleep disorder is sleep apnea. Obstructive sleep apnea (OSA) cases are soon to be crossing the 1 billion mark worldwide [13]. This predominant condition is strongly connected with CV conditions, obesity rates, and several other physical factors; attention on how to best diagnose and manage OSA is vital to providing effective care for OA. OSA is the most common type of sleep apnea and is an obstruction of the airway caused by blockage, narrowing, and decreased musculature, causing the airway to become soft, which is what causes covering of the airway passage [14].

HISTORY

In the older population, both men and postmenopausal women not using hormone replacement therapies (HRT) are affected by OSA at a similar prevalence; it is the most common sleep-breathing disorder [14]. Before menopause, women have protection because of hormone levels of estrogen and progesterone. Postmenopausal women using HRT are provided some protections; however, HRT use is controversial, and the risks and benefits of therapies need further consideration. The use of oral progesterone in men has shown little improvement compared with women [14]. The risk and benefits need to be reviewed per case along with further studies on the matter. OSA is more prevalent in men and women from 30 to 69 years of age; then, there is a plateau in the 70+ age group [15]. The plateau can be attributed to the relationship between body mass index (BMI) and age, which are the significant risk factors for sleep apnea [14,15].

BMI relates to OSA in the general population and shows a stronger indicator for OSA complications with CV conditions. Studies show with increase in weight, and categorizations from normal weight to morbid obesity, there is a correlation of increase in cases of OSA [16]. For OA older than 70 years,

Table 2
Adult sleep disorders

Sleep disorder	Potential causes	Impact on OA
Insomnia A state of hyperarousal that disrupts falling or staying asleep or waking up early & not able to fall back to sleep Can be acute (short term: 1 night to a few weeks); chronic (long term: 3 nights/wk for 3 mo or longer); transient (may come & go) Cannot get enough sleep to feel well rested Most common in the United States Treated with medications, cognitive behavior therapy (CBT), & lifestyle changes	• Poor sleep hygiene • Stress • Irregular sleep schedule • Caffeine (stimulant) • Alcohol (sedative) leading to nonrestorative or fragmented sleep • Medications • Hormonal changes • Mental health disorders (anxiety, depression) • Pain • Traumatic or emotional event • Posttraumatic stress disorder • Neurologic conditions • Physical conditions	• Do not feel well rested when wakening in morning • Exhaustion • Excessive daytime sleepiness • Decreased alertness • Change in mood • Irritability • Decreased memory • Poor performance at work, school, home • Increased errors or accidents • Higher risk of motor vehicle accidents • Decreased quality of life
Narcolepsy A chronic neurologic disorder that impedes the ability of the brain to control sleep-wake cycles Feeling rested after waking but feeling extremely sleepy most of the day; experience interrupted sleep with frequent awakenings during the night major types: Type 1, based on low levels of hypocretin (brain hormone) or reporting cataplexy Type 2, excessive daytime sleepiness but no muscle weakness triggered by emotions; less severe; normal levels of hypocretin Treated with medications & scheduled naps	• Often undiagnosed or misdiagnosed with psychiatric disorders or emotional problems • Low levels of hypocretin • Autoimmune disorders • Family history (up to 10% of diagnoses) • Brain injuries, tumors, or diseases in the area of the brain that regulates wakefulness & REM sleep	• Fall asleep suddenly without warning, often in the middle of doing something, like eating, drinking, writing, driving • Daytime drowsiness • Temporary inability to move or speak (sleep paralysis) just before falling asleep or immediately after waking up • Experience temporary loss of muscle control that leads to feeling weak or limp (cataplexy) • Vivid dreamlike images or hallucinations from wake-to-sleep transition (hypnagogic) or from sleep-to-wake (hypnopompic) transition

(continued on next page)

Table 2 (continued)		
Sleep disorder	Potential causes	Impact on OA
Restless legs syndrome A common neurologic sensory disorder with symptoms produced from within the brain; characterized by unpleasant or uncomfortable sensations in the legs & an uncontrollable urge to move the legs while sitting or lying, especially in the evening Also referred to as Willis-Ekbom disease Symptoms triggered by resting & attempting to sleep Symptoms become more frequent & last longer with aging Treated with medications, CBT, lifestyle changes	• Mainly unknown • Genetic component • Low levels of iron in the brain • Dysfunction of dopamine in the basal ganglia (section of the brain that controls movement), results in involuntary movements • Individuals diagnosed with Parkinson disease • End-stage renal disease; hemodialysis • Medications • Use of alcohol, nicotine, caffeine • Neuropathy	• Exhaustion • Daytime sleepiness • Mood alterations • Lack of ability to concentrate • Inability to carry out daily tasks • Impaired memory • Job, school performance down •Disruption in personal relationships • Contributes to anxiety & depression • Can make traveling difficult

Data from Refs. [9,11,12].

BMI is not a strong indicator because of muscle and weight loss in the 70+ age population [17]. Studies have shown that OA with OSA have a weak association to BMI. It is better to use waist circumference, neck circumference, or a waist-to-hip ratio, which allows for better projecting values. There is a direct relationship of increased fat characteristics in OSA patients, where the upper airway is compromised during sleep because of the body fat surrounding the upper airways, diminishing the full use of the airways, sequentially causing the apneas [17].

The apnea-hypopnea index (AHI) (Fig. 1) is the count of all apneas and hypopneas per hour of sleep, used to classify the disease state and severity:

- 5 to 15 per hour is mild
- 16 to 30 is moderate
- Above 30 is severe [18–21].

Most OA experience heart rate changes during episodes of upper airway obstruction. Obstruction bradycardia is also noted, and during arousal, tachycardia is present. These episodes are typically followed by snoring, oxygen desaturation, and at times, confusion. Because of these episodes, many OA develop excessive daytime sleepiness and require daytime naps to recoup.

Apnea - Hypopnea Index (AHI)		Rating for Sleep Apnea	Apnea Hypopnea Index
• **Apnea** is stops in breathing.		Normal Sleep	Less than events
• **Hypopnea** is moments of shallow breathing.			
• Either one to be counted needs to be at minimum **ten (10) seconds in duration**.		Mild	Between 5 and 15 events
	Moderate	Moderate	Between 15 and 30 events
• AHI calculated by adding all events and dividing by the hours of sleep.	STOP	Severe	More than 30 events

Fig. 1. AHI scale. *Data from* sleepapnea.org/sleep-health-faq.

Once awaken suddenly by apnea, moments tend to lend themselves to nocturia in the OA. Lack of sleep is associated with neurocognitive deficiency, which includes a decline in response time, decline in performance of activities of daily living (ADL), decrease in memory and attention, and places OA at greater risk for falls [17].

ASSESSMENT/PHYSICAL EXAMINATION

Assessment and physical examination (PE) should consist of a full review of body systems with a focus on the head, ears, nose, neck, and throat portions as well as neurocognition. The noted regions of focus should be thoroughly assessed for characteristics that would most likely not be present in other age groups but are reflected in the older population. Starting with the oral cavity allows for visualization of the entire tongue, uvula, tonsils, and soft and hard palates. By having the patient open their mouth, the health care provider (HCP) can observe tongue placement. Fig. 2 depicts the Friedman tongue position stages, which consist of FTP I, FTP IIA, FTP IIb, FTP III, and FTP IV [22].

NPs can visualize the tongue's position with respect to the hard palate, soft palate, uvula base, uvula, and tonsils, along with the relaxed tongue. This staging lends to the start of a combination of assessments in the multisystem testing method. Further assessment includes a health history (HHx) review, which should direct questions toward sleep issues, changes in behaviors, alcohol or tobacco use, and genetic factors [24]. Alcohol affects how the brain controls sleep, especially the muscles involved in breathing and relaxing of muscles, which then affect the closing of the upper airway [24]. Tobacco products, especially smoking/inhalation, cause inflammation and act on how the brain manages sleep and the muscles involved in breathing. Inflammation of the

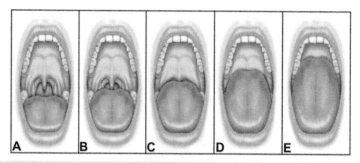

Fig. 2. PE using the Friedman tongue position. (A) FTP I allows visualization of the entire uvula and tonsils/pillars. (B) FTP IIa allows visualization of most of the uvula, but the tonsils/pillars are absent. (C) FTP IIb allows visualization of the entire soft palate to the base of the uvula. (D) In FTP III, some of the soft palate is visualized, but the distal structures are absent. (E) FTP IV allows visualization of the hard palate only [23]. (*From* Friedman M. Friedman tongue position and the staging of obstructive sleep apnea/hypopnea syndrome. In: Sleep Apnea and Snoring: Surgical and Nonsurgical Therapy, Scheidt S, Clansey N (Eds), Philadelphia, Elsevier; 2009; with permission; and Evaluation of the patient with obstructive sleep apnea: Friedman tongue position and staging Author: Michael Friedman, Michelle S. Hwang Publication: Operative Techniques in Otolaryngology-Head and Neck Surgery Publisher: Elsevier; 2015; with permission.)

airways caused by smoking and other associated causes, such as obesity and CV complications, are included as risk factors for OSA [24].

The PE should encompass a review of possible risk factors toward conditions that are problems of sleep apnea (Box 1). Headaches are another hallmark sign of OSA, especially morning headaches that last for several hours upon awakening [25,26]. The headaches are often described as a frontal squeezing without association to nausea or issues with light and sound [25].

The HHx provides a strong foundation to build toward differential diagnoses. Furthermore, an HHx along with a detailed assessment and PE may provide rationales for the occurrences of complications, such as diabetes, arrhythmias, impotence, memory loss, fatigue, changes in behaviors, CV conditions, and other clinical manifestations [27].

DIFFERENTIAL DIAGNOSES

With so many potential complications from OSA, or undiagnosed OSA, sleep issues can present with several similar conditions. For example, the signs and symptoms of gastroesophageal reflux disease can mimic the same as those in a patient with OSA in that they both may have a choking sensation, may have dyspnea at night, and can find benefit from continuous positive airway pressure (CPAP) therapy [28]. Excessive daytime sleepiness is a differential diagnosis that shares a range of the same forms of complications and findings as in OSA. They can be distinguished from the clinical history and polysomnography (or in layman terms, a sleep study), which records the patient's brain waves, records oxygen levels in the blood, monitors heart rate and breathing,

Box 1: Sleep apnea complications
- Memory loss
- Drowsiness
- Fatigue
- Atrial fibrillation
- Heart attack
- Impotence
- Pulmonary hypertension
- Neurologic impairment
- Headache
- Diabetes
- Obesity
- Hypertension
- Stroke
- Falls
- Congestive heart failure
- Cognitive impairment

as well as monitors eye and leg movements during a night spent in a sleep laboratory [24,29]. Other differential diagnoses include asthma, chronic obstructive pulmonary disease (COPD), depression, hypothyroidism, narcolepsy, and periodic limb movement disorders, which share similar findings as excessive daytime sleepiness when a sleep study and testing are completed [30].

DIAGNOSTIC TESTING

NPs can improve the recognition and diagnosis of sleep disorders using screening tools, such as the Epworth Sleepiness Scale (ESS; Fig. 3), collecting sleep histories, and using sleep laboratory tests [31]. Interpretation of results from the ESS uses the following score interpretation [32]:

- 0 to 10 = normal range of sleepiness in healthy adults
- 11 to 14 = mild sleepiness
- 15 to 17 = moderate sleepiness
- 18 to 24 = severe sleepiness

In addition, questionnaires can be used to evaluate if a patient has OSA. Examples of these questionnaires include National Health and Aging Trends Survey questions and the *STOP-Bang* questionnaire, where S represents snoring, T represents tired, O represents observed/stop breathing, P represents pressure, B represents BMI, A represents age older than 50, N represents neck size, and G represents gender [33]. These questionnaires are used to assess risk factors for

---

Epworth Sleepiness Scale

Name: _____ Today's date: _____

Your age (yrs): _____ Your gender (Male = M, Female = F):_____

How likely are you to doze off or fall asleep in the following situations, in contrast to just feeling tired?

This refers to your usual way of life recently. Even if you haven't done some of these things recently, try to figure out how they would have affected you.

Use the following scale to choose the **most appropriate number** for each situation:

> 0 = **no chance** of dozing
> 1 = **slight chance** of dozing
> 2 = **moderate chance** of dozing
> 3 = **high chance** of dozing

It is important that you answer each item as best as you can.

Situation	Chance of Dozing (0-3)
Sitting and reading _____	___
Watching TV _____	___
Sitting inactive in a public place (e.g., a theater or a meeting)	___
As a passenger in a car for an hour without a break _____	___
Lying down to rest in the afternoon when circumstances permit _____	___
Sitting and talking to someone _____	___
Sitting quietly after a lunch without alcohol _____	___
In a car or bus, while stopped for a few minutes in traffic ___	___

THANK YOU FOR YOUR COOPERATION

ESS © MW Johns 1990-1997. Used under License

Fig. 3. ESS. (*From* https://epworthsleepinessscale.com/.)

OSA with a higher yes response equating to more evidence toward a diagnosis of OSA. Further testing includes blood work to check hormone levels and endocrine disorders, and to rule out hypothyroidism, acromegaly, and polycystic ovary syndrome, which can cause sleep apnea [24]. Once a diagnosis of OSA is determined, the patient requires further workup by a sleep specialist, who would order the polysomnography study. Polysomnography encompasses the following:

- Electroencephalogram, which measures the brain waves
- Electro-oculogram, which measures eye movements
- Electromyogram (EMG), which measures muscular activity
- Electrocardiogram, which measures both heart rate and rhythm

- A pulse oximetry test, which monitors the oxygen levels in the blood
- Arterial blood gas analysis [29]

Diagnosis is determined from the presence and frequency of the breathing events during the study.

TREATMENT AND MANAGEMENT

After a positive sleep study, treatment of OSA begins. The first step is for the OA to be fitted for a facial mask, used with a CPAP machine, which is the favored prescribed treatment and most researched machine; this is a first-line therapy [18,22]. There is also bilevel positive airway pressure (BPAP), and autotitrating positive airway pressure (APAP). BPAP offers 2 different pressure levels during the respiratory cycle, typically higher on inspiration and lower during expiration. APAP changes pressure based in response to upper airway airflow resistance. OA that use this form of treatment are found to have COPD or heart failure [18,34]. A major concern for treating OA with positive airway pressure (PAP) devices is adherence to nightly use. Newer technology syncs data directly from PAP devices and logs the usage and interruptions to sleep providing clarification to patient usage. This information is valuable to identify a deeper and more meaningful conversation with the NP. Managing follow-up discussions should include reviewing data recorded by the PAP applications. Management, if not identified through the machine application and the information provided by OA patient, should include a review of medications to see if there are medications that are causing inadequate sleep time. Weight monitoring should be checked at each patient visit; drastic weight changes can affect mask fits, which may cause air leakage in a PAP treatment plan [35].

For those OSA patients who choose or are unable to use a machine, alternative treatments can include a mandibular advancement device, which is worn during sleep. These oral devices have been able to decrease the frequency of sleep events compared with no treatment by shifting the position of the jaw and tongue. The disadvantage for the OA is the need to have good teeth to be able to successfully use an oral appliance [35].

A second option is pharmacologic intervention, and although it is not recommended to be effective enough, includes antimuscarinics and noradrenergic agents. A more natural agent such as cannabis and with many states passing new law toward the use of cannabis, a few studies have shown there is a correlation between use and a decrease in AHI scores when administered 1 hour before bedtime [36]. The NP for OA patients should clearly think about adverse events during the daytime with use of cannabis in the evening and should not currently support use of this pharmacologic treatment until more data and research are accomplished in understanding the full safety spectrum in the OA population. Other pharmacologic therapies, which have not proven to be effective in enough stimulation of the respiratory drive, are theophylline and acetazolamide [30]. With regards to the OA population, all pharmacologic therapies come with more adverse events and are not recommended to implement. The Food and Drug Administration has approved Modafinil, a stimulant, and more recently, in 2019, Solriamfetol, a dopamine/norepinephrine reuptake inhibitor, for the improvement of daytime sleepiness in patients who use a PAP machine routinely but still have remaining sleepiness, preventing the completion of ADL [30].

There are also upper airway surgeries for those who present with abnormalities causing the OSA; however, surgery in the OA patient is not recommended because of adverse effects that may decrease quality of life (QOL) [18,34]. Surgical options include drastic surgeries that come with the risk of surgical complications, including swallowing and voice complications; these include uvulopalatopharyngoplasty, maxillomandibular advancement, tracheostomy, hypoglossal nerve stimulation, radiofrequency reduction of the tongue, stiffening the soft palate with stents, and relocation of bones [18,34]. The current EB treatment is to encourage OA OSA patients to modify their lifestyle to increase positive sleep hygiene practices, lose weight, and use a PAP machine.

IMPLICATIONS FOR NURSE PRACTITIONER PRACTICE

NP, frontline caregivers, need to routinely ask OA about the quality of sleep and screen for OSA [37]. NP should inquire with the OA patient about the quality and daily amount of sleep, and if sleeping is providing the feeling of being refreshed upon awakening. Questioning and discussing sleep practices and sleep hygiene are a vital part of the NP role in working with an OA patient. NP must be mindful in explanations of the importance of sleep at all ages and the use of a polysomnogram test. Explaining the various electrodes that will be attached to the OA and what they are monitoring for is an important factor to discuss with the patient and their family before the testing. Explaining to the patient the electrodes placed near the eyes and on the scalp monitor and record the timing of the different phases of sleep and provide data about REM sleep versus non-REM sleep. Further explanation of electrodes on the chin and jaw line for muscle testing with the EMG complete the technical portion of the conversation [29].

With an understanding of the test, the next concern becomes the cost and the long-term implications if the diagnosis is OSA. The cost to an individual is based on their insurance coverage; however, with more prevalence and reports such as *Hidden Health Crisis Costing America Billions, Underdiagnosing and Undertreating Obstructive Sleep Apnea* by Frost and Sullivan and published in the *American Academy of Sleep Medicine* in 2016, the public and health care professionals are becoming more aware of some of the issues of getting appropriate coverage for certain diagnoses. The report showcases how Medicare and other insurances benefited from providing services for OSA instead of allowing other treatment of the condition. This practice helped to make OSA symptoms become more severe and increase health care costs by the multiple co-morbidities associated with OSA [38]. OSA treatment plans require a CPAP machine, which is covered by most plans. Consideration of the process should be given to families that must go through the routes to document the necessary sleep studies and rule outs for their insurance companies to pay for the study and machine, including the follow-up usage reports, which are programmed into most marketed machines.

NP should be astute when interacting with the OA population, especially when the OA is driving or working with machinery. Drowsy driving or fatigue, owing to OSA, can lead to accidents, including motor vehicle collisions. In the OA population, the increase in falls owing to drowsiness or night awakening episodes from OSA is common; education needs to be provided for fall risk and prevention.

The NP practice should incorporate reviews of EB best practices to maintain and clean the patient's OSA equipment, which may consist of tubing, water reservoirs, and masks. All parts require thorough cleaning and maintenance for longevity.

With the new COVID-19 virus, new information is emerging with recognition that patients with breathing disorders, which include OSA, are at a higher risk for worse outcomes. One reason is due to the comorbidities that are shared between OSA patients and patients who are more susceptible to poor outcomes with COVID-19. These comorbidities include but are not limited to obesity, hypertension, cardiometabolic diseases, diabetes, breathing complications, increases in impaired sleep due to anxiety, depression, and several other disorders that are exacerbated during this pandemic that disturbs healthy sleep hygiene [39,40]. NP should be aware that use of PAP increases the challenges of droplet and aerosol spread. During the ongoing pandemic, HCP taking care of OA diagnosed with OSA need to keep the following in mind:

- Use of telehealth or telemedicine for check-ups
  - As a reminder, not all OA have access to the Internet or technology equipment; telephone calls may be the best way to reach them
- At-home sleep apnea testing
- Using disposable equipment with devices
- Proper personal protective equipment usage
- Use of negative pressure rooms if available [39]

SUMMARY

In review, OA are more prone to OSA because of natural aging-related changes that include decreased musculature tone causing obstructions from weakened airways. An increased amount of body fat around the airways is a major contributing factor to OSA. With OA, weight increases are due in part to body changes from normal aging and metabolism slowing. NP should routinely screen for sleep changes, fall risk assessments, accident assessments, and general overall health of an individual, thus promoting healthy living and evaluating further workup needs for OA patients who may present with OSA symptoms.

OSA is very prevalent in the United States and is highly inappropriately undiagnosed. The US culture often excuses fatigue and drowsiness in the daytime with completing ADL [37]. The most valuable ways to identify OSA are to view the oral cavity and conduct complete detailed assessments and PE while starting with a thorough HHx, including sleep questionnaires. NP should follow up by referral to sleep specialists for further in-depth sleep studies, which may include an overnight stay. Use of index rating sleep and documenting the severity of OSA can then be discriminated toward and separated out from differential diagnoses.

The next step would be treatment and management of the sleep apnea pressure therapies. Using PAP therapy and living a healthy lifestyle include the following:

- Maintaining a healthy weight
- Engaging in regular physical activities
- Limiting alcohol and tobacco usage
- Creating a healthy sleep environment
- Ensuring appropriate sleep hygiene is practiced routinely for gaining adequate hours of restful sleep

The NP should encourage OSA CPAP users to maintain and clean their devices routinely to prevent illness because of unsanitized equipment.

Sleep hygiene, healthy life choices, losing weight, and maintaining a healthy weight to prevent airway obstructions due to body fat are vital for the OA to decrease apnea episodes. When using a PAP machine continuously for a 1-month duration, positive reversal in OSA patients has been documented related to intrinsic physiology changes [41]. The importance of sleep, understanding one's personal sleep requirements, and maintaining the ability to perform at one's peak performance level, at any age, are vital.

The contributing factors listed previously will help reinforce the imperative need for sleep hygiene and healthy lifestyle choices. NP conversations with OA should highlight that with adequate sleep, the mind-body-spirit can be refreshed to improve QOL. OSA patients should also be provided education for fall prevention, which allows the OA to keep as independent as possible for as long as possible. Isn't that what all clinicians want for their OA patients?

CLINICS CARE POINTS

- Questioning and discussing sleep practices and sleep hygiene are vital parts of the examination.
- Routinely screen patients for sleep changes, fall risk, accidents, and overall health assessments including comorbidities.
- Monitor age-related changes in musculature tone and weakened airways.
- For those using CPAP type machines for treatment review usage, maintenance, and all concerns for adherence.

References

[1] National Sleep Foundation. 25 random facts about sleep. 2020. Available at: https://www.sleepfoundation.org/articles/25-random-facts-about-sleep. Accessed June 18, 2020.

[2] National Sleep Foundation. How excessive sleep can affect your metabolism. 2020. Available at: https://www.sleepfoundation.org/articles/how-excessive-sleep-can-affect-yourmetabolism.

[3] Hirshkowitz M, Whiton K, Albert SM, et al. National Sleep Foundation's sleep time duration recommendations: methodology and results summary. Sleep Health 2015;1:40–3.

[4] Centers for Disease Control and Prevention. Short sleep duration among US adults. 2017. Available at: https://www.cdc.gov/sleep/data_statistics.html.

[5] Centers for Disease Control and Prevention. Perceived insufficient rest or sleep among adults - United States. MMWR Morb Mortal Wkly Rep 2008;58:1179.

[6] Abraham O, Pu J, Schleiden LJ, et al. Factors contributing to poor satisfaction with sleep and healthcare seeking behavior in older adults. Sleep Health 2017;3:43–8.

[7] Li J, Vitiello MV, Gooneratne NS. Sleep in normal aging. Sleep Med Clin 2018;13(1): 1–11.

[8] Centers for Disease Control and Prevention. Tips for better sleep.. 2016. Available at: https://www.cdc.gov/sleep/about_sleep/sleep_hygiene.html.

[9] National Institutes of Health. United States National Library of Medicine. Sleep disorders. 2018. Available at: https://medlineplus.gov/sleepdisorders.html#.

[10] American Sleep Association. Sleep and sleep disorder statistics. 2018. Available at: https://www.sleepassociation.org/about-sleep/sleep-statistics/.

[11] Center for Disease Control and Prevention. Sleep and sleep disorders. 2020. Available at: https://www.cdc.gov/sleep/index.html.

[12] Wolkove N, Elkholy O, Baltzan M, et al. Sleep and aging:1. Sleep disorders commonly found in older people. Can Med Assoc J 2007;176(9):1299–304.

[13] Garbarina S, Magnavita M, Sanna A, et al. Estimating the hidden burden of obstructive sleep apnea: challenges and pitfalls. Lancet Respir Med 2020;8(1); https://doi.org/10.101016/S2213-2600(19)304163.

[14] Bixler EO, Vgontzas AN, Lin HM, et al. Prevalence of sleep-disordered breathing in women: effects of gender. Am J Respir Crit Care Med 2001;163:608.

[15] Benjafield AV, Ayas NT, Eastwood PR, et al. Estimation of the global prevalence and burden of obstructive sleep apnea: a literature-based analysis. Lancet Respir Med 2019;7:687.

[16] Tufik S, Santos-Silva R, Taddei JA, et al. Obstructive sleep apnea syndrome in the Sao Paulo Epidemiologic Sleep Study. Sleep Med 2010;11:441.

[17] Lee Y-JG, Jeong DU. Differential effects of obesity on obstructive sleep apnea syndrome according to age. Psychiatry Investig 2017;14(5):656–61. Available at: https://www.ncbi.nlm.nih.gov/pmc/articles/PMC5639134/#.

[18] AHI Scale. Created by. Nina Ganesh Nandish, AGPCNP-BC 2020. Original figures/tables using previously published data. Available at: https://www.sleepapnea.org/sleep-health-faq.

[19] Clip Art, (Stop) C:\Users\Nina\AppData\Local\Microsoft\Windows\Temporary Internet Files\Content.IE5\X1UWBITO\1024px-Iceland_road_sign_B19.11.svg[1].png.

[20] Clip Art, (Moderate) C:\Users\Nina\AppData\Local\Microsoft\Windows\Temporary Internet Files\Content.IE5\D9XPBWQN\moderate[1].jpg.

[21] Clip Art, (Thumbs up) C:\Users\Nina\AppData\Local\Microsoft\Windows\Temporary Internet Files\Content.IE5\LH5R6DK1\1024px-Thumb_up_icon.svg[1].png.

[22] Friedman M. Friedman tongue position and the staging of obstructive sleep apnea/hypopnea syndrome. In: Scheidt S, Clansey N, editors. Sleep apnea and snoring: surgical and nonsurgical therapy. Philadelphia: Elsevier; 2009.

[23] Friedman M, Michelle S. Evaluation of the patient with obstructive sleep apnea: Friedman tongue position and staging. Hwang Publication: Operative Techniques in Otolaryngology-Head and Neck Surgery Publisher: Elsevier Inc; 2015.

[24] National Institutes of Health, National Institutes of Health Sleep Disorders Research Plan. Available at: https://www.nhlbi.nih.gov/node/4228 https://www.nhlbi.nih.gov/health-topics/sleep-studies.

[25] Russell MB, Kristiansen HA, Kvaerner KJ. Headache in sleep apnea syndrome: epidemiology and pathophysiology. Cephalalgia 2014;34:752.

[26] Sleep Apnea Complications Slide Created by. Nina Ganesh Nandish, AGPCNP-BC 2020.

[27] American Sleep Apnea Association, 2000 Pennsylvania Avenue NW, #7000 Washington, DC 20006. Available at: https://www.sleepapnea.org/ufaqs/what-is-ahi-represent/.

[28] Tawk M, Goodrich S, Kinasewitz G, et al. The effect of 1 week of continuous positive airway pressure treatment in obstructive sleep apnea patients with concomitant gastroesophageal reflux. Chest 2006;130:1003.

[29] Available at: https://www.healthline.com/health/sleep/obstructive-sleep-apnea

[30] Available at: https://emedicine.medscape.com/article/295807-differential and medication.

[31] Winkelman JW. Screening for Excessive Daytime Sleepiness and Diagnosing Narcolepsy. J Clin Psychiatry 2020;81(4):HB19045BR1C. Available at: https://www.psychiatrist.com/JCP/article/Pages/2020/v81/HB19045BR1C.aspx.

[32] Dr Johns' personal website about the ESS. Available at: http://epworthsleepinessscale.com/ ESS © MW Johns 1990-1997. Questionnaire used with the permission of Mapi Research Trust, 27 rue de la Villette, 69003 Lyon, France. Graphic ESS - United States/English - Version of 19 Jan 18 - Mapi. ID037309/ESS_AU1.0_eng-US2.doc.

[33] Chung F, Yegneswaran B, Liao P, et al. STOP questionnaire: a tool to screen patients for obstructive sleep apnea. Anesthesiology 2008;108:812–21. Available at: https://anesthesiology.pubs.asahq.org/article.aspx?articleid=1932315.

[34] Lee-Chiong TL. Obstructive sleep apnea disrupts elders' sleep. Todays Geriatr Med 2015;8(2): 26. Available at: https://www.todaysgeriatricmedicine.com/archive/0315p26.shtml.

[35] Available at: http://healthysleep.med.harvard.edu/sleep-apnea/diagnosing-osa/understanding-results#:~:text=obstructive%20sleep%20apnea.-,Apnea%20Hypopnea%20Index%20(AHI),Minimal%3A%20AHI%20%3C%205%20per%20hour produced by WGBH Educational Foundation for the Harvard Medical School Division of Sleep Medicine (DSM) as one activity of the Sleep and Health Education Program. Understanding Sleep (TM), Get Sleep (TM), and Got Sleep (TM) are trademarks of the President and Fellows of Harvard College.

[36] Carley DW, Prasad B, Reid KJ, et al. Pharmacotherapy of apnea by cannabimimetic enhancement, the PACE clinical trial: effects of dronabinol in obstructive sleep apnea. Sleep 2018;41:zsx184.

[37] Available at: https://aasm.org/resources/pdf/sleep-apnea-economic-crisis.pdf

[38] Hidden Health Crisis Costing America Billions. Underdiagnosing and undertreating obstructive sleep apnea draining healthcare system. Darien (IL): American Academy of Sleep Medicine; 2016.

[39] Voulgaris A, Ferini-Strambi L, Steiropoulos P. Sleep medicine and COVID-19. Has a new era begun? [published online ahead of print, 2020 Jul 17]. Sleep Med 2020;73:170–6.

[40] Feuth T, Saaresranta T, Karlsson A, et al. Is sleep apnoea a risk factor for COVID-19? Findings from a retrospective cohort study. medRxiv 2020; https://doi.org/10.1101/2020.05.14.20098319.

[41] Edwards BA, Wellman A, Sands SA, et al. Obstructive sleep apnea in older adults is a distinctly different physiological phenotype. Sleep 2014;37(7):1227–36.

Assessment and Management of Constipation in Older Adults

Linda J. Keilman, DNP, GNP-BC[a],*,
Katherine Dontje, PhD, FNP-BC[b]

[a]Michigan State University, College of Nursing, 1355 Bogue Street, A126 Life Science Building, East Lansing, MI 48824-1317, USA; [b]Michigan State University, College of Nursing, 1355 Bogue Street, A118 Life Science Building, East Lansing, MI 48824-1317, USA

Keywords

• Constipation • Older adult • Bowel movement • Interventions for constipation

Key points

• Constipation is not a normal condition of aging. Although it is more frequent in older adults, there generally are effective lifestyle changes that can be made to alleviate the condition.

• Constipation generally is not the chief complaint of patients in primary care.

• The advanced practice registered nurse (APRN) needs to understand constipation is common and not an easy subject for older adults to discuss and thus incorporate defecation questions in review of systems for all patients.

• The best way to treat constipation is to prevent constipation. This requires a holistic proactive approach to patients by the APRN.

INTRODUCTION

Foundational nursing programs introduce students to every human body system. Remember learning about the gastrointestinal (GI) system? Bowel movements (BMs), bowel patterns, toileting habits, incontinence, types, amount, shapes (forms), colors, consistency, size, and smell? Who knew there was so much to know about one bodily function that is basically how digested food and fluids become stool/feces and moves through the mouth to the rectum and out of the body? Nursing students generally are taught that older adults (OAs) can be fixated on their bowels. After certifying as a gerontological nurse practitioner, the authors realized that BM

*Corresponding author. E-mail address: keilman@msu.edu

https://doi.org/10.1016/j.yfpn.2021.01.003
2589-420X/21/© 2021 Elsevier Inc. All rights reserved.

fixation (or preoccupation) is common in OAs. There is much GI knowledge providers need in order to help OAs maintain social engagement, perform activities of daily living, maintain their desired quality of life (QOL), and prevent constipation. In this article, the authors briefly describe basic constipation in OAs that primary care providers (PCPs) need to understand: prevalence, definitions, types, basic pathophysiology, assessment, diagnosis, and treatment–including education and referral.

PREVALENCE AND COST

Constipation is a symptom leading to a common GI disorder, resulting in more than 3 million yearly visits to PCPs [1]. These visits generally are not the chief complaint (CC) but often come up in the history or review of systems (ROS), during over-the-counter (OTC) medication or home remedies review, or just as the PCP is leaving the room after concluding the visit. If constipation is the CC, the visit is not necessarily evaluated in a holistic or systematic process. In many cases, the OA perception of constipation and the actual diagnosis are not consistent. Constipation refers to the symptoms an individual is experiencing related to defecation. Basically, the general (non–health care–educated) population in this country do not fully understand facts about BMs–especially what is normal or a deviation from normal. Therein lies one of the reasons that constipation is a frequent issue in the OA population. One in 5 OAs has constipation issues at some point in their lives [2]. Constipation, however, is not a normal part of aging.

Constipation increases with age. A current estimate of constipation in community-dwelling OAs is between 6% and 18%; in long-term care settings, the estimate is greater than 60% to 70% of OAs [3]. Women are more prone than men to live with constipation until their mid-60s–then the percentage for both genders levels out. Prevalence peaks after age 70. It also is well known in gerontology/geriatric services that the prevalence of constipation is underestimated by OAs and PCPs and, therefore, is under-recognized and undertreated.

The impact of constipation on health care expenditures and QOL is burdensome. During 2017 to 2018, the British National Health Service spent approximately $162 million on treating constipation across the life span [4]. In the United States, cost of constipation care includes emergency department visits (approximately 700,000 in 2017), constipation primary diagnosis admissions to hospitals, consultations, investigations, and OTC laxatives [5,6]. Approximately $82 million are spent annually in the United States on laxatives [6]. Approximately 75% of individuals living in long-term care take at least 1 laxative daily [6]. Although financially expensive and a significant factor in the US National Health Expenditure 2019 data [7], constipation has an impact on an individuals' mental, physical, emotional, social, and spiritual dimensions and is of great significance to the OA population. Constipation also has a negative impact on OAs still in the workforce as well as preventing them from being socially engaged in their communities.

DEFINITION AND TYPES

The definitions of constipation can vary greatly, especially when comparing/contrasting by a PCP versus by a gastroenterologist. Diagnosis of constipation is based on symptoms and is somewhat subjective. The most common definition of constipation is infrequent BMs or difficulty passing stool that lasts for several weeks or longer. Another description is having less than 3 BMs in 1 week. Many Americans believe they need to have a daily BM. Although that may be the usual pattern for some individuals, it is not the majority defecation pattern. Many OAs define constipation as straining in order to evacuate their bowels. The more frail and older an individual is, the more likely they are to develop constipation. This is related to a variety of issues, including decreased physical activity, immobility, poor nutrition (lack of daily fresh fruits, vegetables, and fiber), dehydration from lack of fluid intake, and polypharmacy. Constipation also is more common in aging living environments (adult foster care, assisted living, nursing homes, etc) and during hospitalizations. Bottom line, the goal for constipation in OAs is based on the PCP history and examination considering defecation frequency and patient comfort level. Constipation may be acute–symptoms last less than 1 week and generally are preceded by a change in daily routine or lifestyle. Chronic constipation is defecation issues that have been present for a minimum of 3 months.

Constipation in OAs often is associated with chronic comorbid conditions, including lower urinary tract symptoms, overflow fecal incontinence [6], fecal impaction, intestinal obstruction, and exacerbation of neurodegenerative diseases, such as Alzheimer disease or Parkinson disease–to name a few. Additionally, OAs who strain to move their bowels are at risk for development of hemorrhoids (both internal and external), anal fissures, and rectal prolapse.

Risk factors for constipation include

- Older age
- Female gender
- Dehydration
- Low fiber and low caloric intake
- Physical inactivity
- Immobility
- Certain medications (eg, sedatives, antacids with calcium, iron supplements, opioid pain medications, antidepressants, and hypertensive meds); polypharmacy
- Lower socioeconomic status
- Less formal education
- Diagnosed/living with a mental health issue (depression, anxiety, or eating disorder)

Constipation can be divided into primary (functional or idiopathic) and secondary, which generally is caused by specific medication use and chronic conditions. Symptoms for constipation include

- Going without a BM for more than 3 days

- Less than 3 BMs/wk
- Straining/pushing to start or complete a BM
- Consistency of feces that resemble nuts, rocks, or small pebbles
- Hard consistency
- Needing to manually remove stool from the rectum
- After leaving the toilet, feeling there has not been complete emptying

A functional constipation diagnosis is derived from a complete health history, appropriate physical examination, and, if indicated, limited testing (eg, colonoscopy) [8]. More information is discussed later.

Primary or simple constipation occurs when there is a malfunction of the defecation process or intrinsic defects in colonic function [8]. The types of functional/idiopathic constipation are presented in Box 1. Terminology utilized for the specific type generally is what information is needed in primary care. More complicated constipation should be referred to a GI specialty practice for definitive diagnosis.

Constipation falls into the category of functional GI disorders, which are defined as disorders of gut-brain interaction [10,11]. The Rome IV diagnostic criteria categorize 4 subtypes of chronic constipation: (1) functional constipation (7.8%), (2) irritable bowel syndrome (IBS) with constipation (4.6%), (3) opioid-induced constipation (1.5%), and (4) functional defecation disorders—bloating (3.1%) and diarrhea (4.7%) [12,13]. Percentages indicate the prevalence of functional bowel disorders in adults (1 out of 4) in the United States, Canada, and the United Kingdom [13]. Beginning in 1978, the Rome dynamic process and criteria were developed by global functional GI disorders experts for research; starting with criteria III, adaptations to the diagnostic criteria were made so they could be utilized in primary care [14]. The Rome IV criteria were updated in 2016 [15]. Each of these types has various causes and treatments. Thus, it is important to do a systematic review and analysis of the OA patient's symptoms.

ASSESSMENT

The most important aspect of the overall assessment is learning the person's individual story, which requires asking meaningful and appropriate questions and attentive listening. Every individual is different—a unique human being. As such, it is imperative to understand where a person has come from—this information can be captured by asking about their social determinants of health (SDOHs). Why collect OA patient data via SDOHs? SDOHs can account for up to 40% of patient outcomes [16], especially among marginalized, vulnerable, and minority populations. Additionally, SDOHs are the conditions in which people are born, grow, live, work, and age. Differences in community and national distribution of money, power, and resources in a person's life can lead to health inequities and disparities [17]. Health inequities and disparities can result in decreased QOL, lack of access and quality in their health care, health illiteracy, lack of holistic self-care practices, and decreased esteem and well-being [18] (Fig. 1).

Box 1: Functional constipation types

Type	Characteristics	Patient report	Pearls

Normal transit	• Most common
	• Stool moves through the intestine at usual or normal rate
	• Reduced colon transit cannot be confirmed
	• Some patients may have
	  o Increased rectal compliance
	  o Reduced rectal sensation
	  o OR both
	• Overlaps with IBS with constipation [3]
	• Patient reported
		• Feeling constipated
		• Patient perception
		• Difficulty with evacuation
		• Bloating
		• Abdominal pain
		• Feeling uncomfortable
		• Hard stools
		• Increased psychosocial stress
			• Provide patient with BM diary × 2 wk
			• Follow-up in clinic in 3 wk
			• Fiber supplementation beneficial
			• Usually responds to fiber supplementation, increased fluid and possible short-term use of laxatives

Slow transit	• Prolonged intestinal transit time (colon) or reduced motility of the large intestine
	• Impairment of propulsive colonic motor activity
	• Diminished colonic responses following a meal and on awakening in the morning
	• Impaired colonic motor response to cholinergic stimulation in descending colon
	• May be caused by enteric nerve abnormalities
		• Frequent stools
		• Loose stools
		• Abdominal pain
		• Bloating
		• Soiling of underwear and clothing
		• Fear/embarrassment about loss of bowel control, especially outside the home
		• Depression
		• Decreased self-esteem
		• Social isolation
			• Educate the patient on the 3 Fs [9]:
			  o Fluid
			  o Fruit
			  o Fiber
			• If constipated for some time, may want to start with a laxative to get the GI system working
			• Electrical stimulation

Pelvic floor dysfunction	• Inability to relax and coordinate pelvic floor muscles to have a BM • Difficulty evacuating stool/feces • Urine or stool that leaks	• Straining to defecate • Incomplete emptying of the bowel • Constipation • Female pain during intercourse • Male erectile dysfunction	• Pelvic floor exercises done appropriately • Kegel trainer • Weight management • Biofeedback (retrain muscles) [9]

(continued on next page)

(continued)

Type	Characteristics	Patient report	Pearls

	• Some common causes:
	  ○ Traumatic injury
	  ○ Heredity
	  ○ Pregnancy
	  ○ Pelvic surgery
	  ○ Nerve damage
	  ○ Advancing age
	  ○ Overweight or obesity
	  ○ Pushing/straining over time
		• Urine or fecal incontinence
		• Urinary frequency
		• Frequent urinary tract infections
			• Physical therapy
			• Keep stools soft

A history and physical examination should be performed in OAs with constipation to identify alarm features or symptoms. OAs should be asked if they have unexplained fever, unintentional weight loss, blood in the stool, vomiting, and abdominal pain. Other concerning features are individuals who are over age 50 and have recent onset of symptoms or are diagnosed with iron deficiency anemia. The causes of some of these symptoms could be colon cancer,

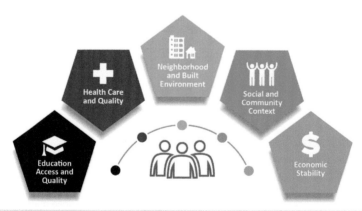

Fig. 1. CDC—SDOHs. CDC stacks is a free, digital archive of scientific research and literature produced by the Centers for Disease Control and Prevention and is within the public domain. Accessed December 20, 2020. https://www.cdc.gov/publichealthgateway/sdoh/index.html.

tumor, rectocele, or diverticulosis–to name a few. An additional correlation with constipation is cognitive impairment/dementia, depression, autonomic neuropathy, or Parkinson disease.

A person's story and individual SDOHs can be captured through an evaluation that includes the CC, history of present illness (HPI), ROS, family medical history (FMH), past medical history (PMH), past surgical history (PSH), social history (SocH), and medications. Table 1 describes specifics for each category.

The Bristol stool scale, originally developed in 1997, classifies stool/feces into 7 different categories. Types 1 and 2 indicate constipation; types 3 and 4 are considered the gold standard or ideal stools because they are soft and easier to pass; and types 5 through 7 may indicate diarrhea and urgency [19]. Show the patient the chart and have them pick which type looks like their BMs.

PHYSICAL EXAMINATION
After the subjective information is collected in the history, it is important to gather objective information through a focused PE. Components to assess are found in Box 2.

DIAGNOSIS
Depending on a patient's clinical presentation, history, and PE, it may be important to do additional diagnostic testing. Blood work is not cost-effective or recommended routinely, however, without presence of alarm features [21]. Plain abdominal imaging studies have poor evidence and there is a lack of standardization and controlled studies for use in primary care [21]. Also not routinely recommended are barium enema studies related to radiation exposure and lack of controlled studies [21]. There are several physiologic tests that can help to determine the cause of constipation, including (1) colonic transit study, (2) anorectal manometry, and (3) balloon expulsion test [6]. This type of testing generally is outside of primary care and reserved for patients with abnormal findings and who do not respond to symptomatic treatment [14]. Further explanation of these diagnostic tests is outside the focus of this article.

MANAGEMENT AND TREATMENT
Once a diagnosis of constipation has been determined, the next step is the type of constipation. The PCP and patient mutually can determine the most appropriate treatment plan through a shared decision-making process. The first step is to educate the patient as to what constipation is and encourage them to try lifestyle changes. Lifestyle changes include increasing fiber and fluids as well as physical activity. The American Society of Colon and Rectal Surgeons indicates that the use of fiber and fluids as first-line interventions is a strong recommendation based on moderate-quality evidence [22]. Even though the evidence

Table 1
Components of the patient defecation history

Specific portion	Areas to specifically address related to defecation issues
CC Specific toward difficulties with defecation	• Using the patient's words (quote) is very important • Do not alter their words • Document exactly what is said • Use quotation marks, so evident that the comment is the patient's words
HPI Including cardinal features of the symptom	• Temporal characteristics: When did it start (onset)? How long has it been going on (duration)? What has happened over time? Constant or intermittent? • Location: this characteristic is important if the patient is describing pain; determining where is very important (back; perineum; vagina; testicles; pubic region; abdomen; inguinal region) • Intensity: severity of difficulty with defecation; how is the patient bothered by what is going on; if there is pain, use a visual analog or verbal scale (If 0 is no pain and 10 is the worst pain imaginable, what number is the pain?); document what the patient verbalizes • Quality: What is the nature of the issue? Does constipation interfere with work life; social life; well-being; self-esteem? • Aggravating factors: history of precipitating events; Has there been any change in food or fluid intake? New medication? Physical activity decreased? Issues with mobility; Stress; Change in what eating or drinking? • Alleviating factors: this is the place to determine whether the patient has been using enemas, laxatives or manipulation—For how long? How do they get relief? • Related symptoms: bloating (feeling of fullness); cramping; flatulence (gas); eructation (belching or burping; voluntary or involuntary); hematochezia (vomiting of blood; coffee ground appearance); Any recent weight loss—especially more than 10 lb (4.5 kg)? • What does the patient think it is: by asking the patient's opinion, this is where the PCP finds out a lot about what the patient is thinking or feeling; the patient might offer a lot of information here as well—often related to HPI questions or ROS; some OAs are fearful they may have cancer or another chronic disease; empathy and sensitivity are important in this questioning.
ROS	• Lifetime history of stool frequency, consistency, need to strain, use of perineal maneuvers during defecation (pushing on perineum, gluteal region, rectovaginal wall, leaning forward on the toilet, raising feet on a stool) • Prolonged straining • Digital evacuation • Feel urge to defecate—respond immediately or wait? • Satisfaction after defecation • Use of laxative or enema: frequency, type, results • How much time spent on toilet per BM • Presence/amount of blood in stool; frequency • History of sigmoidoscopy or colonoscopy

(continued on next page)

Table 1 (continued)	
Specific portion	Areas to specifically address related to defecation issues
	• Usual BM pattern (no. in a wk)
	• Usual bowel habits (time of day; how long spend in bathroom; privacy)
	• Use the Bristol stool scale for stool/feces specifics (Fig. 2)
	• Nausea, vomiting
	• Presence of urinary incontinence with activity
FMH	• Bowel function and GI disease
	• Cancer
	• Chronic diseases: cardiovascular, diabetes, hypertension, hyperlipidemia, renal
	• Neurogenic conditions
	• Psychogenic conditions (depression, anxiety, and somatization)
	• Hereditary/genetic disease
	• Mental health issues
	• Family ancestry
PMH	• Childhood illness
	• Adult illness
	• Childbirth: babies' weight; number; vaginal or cesarean section delivery; with or without forceps or episiotomy
PSH	• Type, date, where surgical procedure accomplished
	• Specifically: GI tract, abdominal, renal, genitourinary, back
SocH	• Living environment: growing up; rural vs urban; current arrangements; live alone or with others; feel safe in community
	• Location of bathrooms in living environment
	• Highest level of education
	• Reading ability
	• Work history: lifelong and current
	• Health insurance
	• 24-h food and fluid intake; Is this usual pattern? ask about breakfast, lunch, dinner, snacks; ask specifically about water and fiber intake.
	• Able to shop for groceries; ability to prepare and cook meals
	• Alcohol use: specific type; amount; how often; how long
	• Caffeine: amount; how often; how long; type
	• Smoking: cigarettes, cigars, pipe; chewing tobacco; vaping (inhaling a vapor created by an e-cigarette or vaping device)
	• Use of marijuana, cocaine, heroin, opioids or other drugs: specifics; frequency; how long
	• Physical activity
	• Hobbies/interests
	• Marital/relationship status; sexually active
	• [a] How does culture or ethnicity have an impact on health?
	• [a] Is there anything I (PCP) need to know in order to take respectful care of you?
	• [a] How do you get through difficult times?
	o This may help define faith, spirituality, complementary and alternative medicine practices; support system

(continued on next page)

Table 1 (continued)	
Specific portion	Areas to specifically address related to defecation issues

Medications	• Laxatives: type, number, and frequency
	• Enemas: type, number, and frequency
	• Prescription medication: name, route, dose, frequency, how long, and what taking for
	• OTC: list all but may want to specifically ask about the following:
	  ○ Herbal laxative: Senna glycoside (oral, rectal forms; contains glycosides, which stimulate gut innervation and increase colonic transit time)
	  ○ Osmotic laxative: magnesium citrate (pulls water into the intestines, mixes with dry feces, leading to easier expulsion; ask about amount of water intake if taking this medication)
	  ○ Probiotics—bifidobacteria, lactobacillus (live bacteria occurring in the gut; increase stool frequency and consistency
	  ○ Flaxseed oil
	• Home remedies: a medication or tonic administered without a prescription or professional supervision; not evidence-based; generally passed down in the family; may be cultural

a Not traditional SocH questions; however, they provide information related to culture/ethnic beliefs that may have an impact on bowel patterns; how best to collaborate with the patient and mutually determine plans of care; and understanding how important faith/spirituality are in OAs' lives.

is moderate, it is important that OA patients understand that healthy habits may help with constipation.

Dietary fiber intake is the first line, with a recommendation of 25 g of fiber per day. This seems simple but only a small percentage of individuals consume this amount of fiber daily. For those attempting to increase their fiber, it should be done gradually to prevent side effects, such as gaseousness. The expected outcome of increasing fiber is to increase the frequency and bulk of the stool. Up to 85% of individuals with no pathologic reason for constipation respond to fiber treatment [22]. There are 2 types of fiber—soluble and insoluble. Soluble fiber increases the bulk of stools and insoluble fiber increases the speed stool moves through the intestine. Both are important in a healthy diet, but soluble fiber has been found more beneficial to improve symptoms of constipation [23]. Probiotics have been presented as an option, but few studies have been done to determine efficacy [24].

Lifestyle changes often are recommended for improvement of constipation but there is little evidence to support these interventions [25]. Even with this in mind, it is important the patient understand that healthy habits may help with constipation. A healthy lifestyle is paramount in the lives of OAs in order to stay engaged in life and increase their QOL.

Box 2: Components of the physical examination

- General appearance
- Vital signs: temperature; pulse; respirations; blood pressure
- Height; weight; body mass index
- Orientation
- Skin: tenting; texture; presence of ecchymosis, skin tears
- Neuro: sensation, strength, reflexes; may find signs of systemic disease that may cause constipation
- Lymph node palpation in upper torso and inguinal region
- Abdomen: detailed examination
  - Inspection: scars, striae, vascular changes, protrusions; general contour
  - Auscultation: all 4 quadrants; normal is gurgling bowel sounds every 5 seconds to 10 seconds; listen for bruits
  - Percussion: determine size and location of intra-abdominal organs; all 4 quadrants; normal is tympanic sounds over air-filled stomach/intestinal quadrants; muffled sounds over fluid-filled or solid organs (eg, liver or spleen)
  - Superficial palpation
  - Deep palpation: all 4 quadrants; assess intra-abdominal organs for potential signs of peritonitis
    - Rebound tenderness: increase in pain caused by irritation of the receptors in the parietal peritoneum
    - Abdominal guarding: contraction of the abdominal wall muscles
      - Rigidity: involuntary guarding; tightening of muscles due to peritoneal inflammation; generally localized to a specific quadrant
      - Voluntary guarding: voluntary contraction to avoid pain during examination; over the entire abdomen
  - Palpation of the liver or spleen
- Anal orifice: inspect of anus and surrounding tissue; excoriation, scars, fissures, masses, tags, lesions, prolapse, hemorrhoids, sphincter tone; perineal sensation—check for anal wink reflex
- Digital rectal examination: palpate for anorectal strictures [12]; rectal bleeding, prostate evaluation [20]; sensation; strength of resting sphincter tone; squeeze maneuver—ask patient to squeeze and hold for up to 30 seconds (normal, decreased, or increased)
  - Pushing and bearing down maneuver: finger in rectum, hand on patient's abdomen to assess push effort; ask patient to push and bear down as if to defecate [21].

The second recommended treatment is osmotic laxatives, such as polyethylene glycol and lactulose. The evidence related to osmotic laxatives is moderate quality [22]. These supplements draw fluid into the bowel to increase the water in the stool and assist with propulsion. Side effects are increase in gas and occasional nausea with lactulose [26]. Stimulant laxatives, such as

Type 1		Separate hard lumps, like nuts (hard to pass)
Type 2		Sausage-shaped but lumpy
Type 3		Like a sausage, but with cracks on the surface
Type 4		Like a sausage or snake, smooth and soft
Type 5		Soft blobs with clear-cut edges (passed easily)
Type 6		Fluffy pieces with ragged edges, a mushy stool
Type 7		Watery, no solid pieces (entirely liquid)

Fig. 2. The Bristol stool form scale. Creative commons attribution. Masaki Maruyama, Kenya Kamimura, Moeno Sugita, Nao Nakajima, Yoshifumi Takahashi, Osamu Isokawa and Shuji Terai (January 9th 2019). The Management of Constipation: Current Status and Future Prospects, Constipation, Gyula Mózsik, IntechOpen, https://doi.org/10.5772/intechopen.83467. Available from: https://www.intechopen.com/books/constipation/the-management-of-constipation-current-status-and-future-prospects.

bisacodyl and Senna glycoside, often are the next option. These medications are proved to increase colonic contractions; however, few studies have been done on these medications [6]. Those studies that have been done show no safety issues with long-term use [26].

If these recommendations have not been effective within 30 days, the next step is to place an OA patient on intestinal secretagogues. These include lubiprostone, linaclotide, and plecanatide, all of which are approved by the Food and Drug Administration for treating chronic constipation. Each of these medications works slightly differently. Lubiprostone increases fluid secretion and improves small bowel transit. Lubiprostone is approved for treatment of chronic constipation, opioid-induced constipation, and IBS with constipation. Linaclotide and plecanatide are approved for IBS with constipation and for chronic constipation. Linaclotide impacts the chloride channel and pulls water into the intestinal lumen. Plecanatide is a guanylyl cyclase C agonist and works in a similar way to lubiprostone to increase intestinal fluid; some studies show it may have an impact on visceral hypersensitivity to improve abdominal pain [22,23]. Patients who are refractory to these treatments should be referred for further testing to determine anorectal physiology and colon transit investigation.

IMPLICATIONS FOR PRACTICE

Freedom of the bowels is the most precious, perhaps even the most essential, of all freedoms—one without which little can be accomplished.

—Émile Gautier, 1909 [8]

Prevention and treatment of constipation should be priorities for every OA cared for by an advanced practice registered nurse (APRN). The best clinical practice to follow is to be proactive and question every adult and OA patient about their bowel habits and patterns. Talking about bowels in many cases is embarrassing and not something usually discussed with other people–including PCPs. It is up to APRNs to understand that constipation is common in OAs although not a part of normal aging. And, because constipation generally is not the reason for a PC visit, it is up to the APRN to make it a habit to ask routine questions about BMs. In most cases, a focused approach to the CC of the unique patient reveals easy lifestyle interventions that can be discussed through education–verbally and in writing. Empathizing with OAs and understanding the impact of the condition on their lives help create a therapeutic relationship where mutual shared decision making is successful and expected health outcomes are reached.

CLINICS CARE POINTS

- There is a misconception related to bowel movements, especially with older adults and what is considered normal. Exact questioning must be used when talking with patients to determine what their unique bowel patterns are in order to diagnose deviations.
- Over-the counter medications for constipation are often highlighted in magazines and in television commercials. Asking direct questions about use of these products (laxatives, suppositories, enemas, fiber, etc.) is extremely important when trying to return the bowel to a drug-free system.
- The introduction of fiber into a daily routine that is void of fiber must be accomplished at a slow, stepped pace in order to not overwhelm the intestinal tract.
- Individuals must first be taught how the bowel functions, what is considered "normal". and how lifestyle changes and nutrition/hydration can lead to positive outcomes.

Disclosure

Authors have nothing to disclose.

References

[1] Dimidi E, Cox C, Grant R, et al. Perceptions of constipation among the general public and people with constipation differ strikingly from those of general and specialist doctors and the Rome IV criteria. Am J Gastroenterol 2019;114(7):1116–29.
[2] Lee L. Constipation: causes and prevention tips. John Hopkins Medicine. 2020. Available at: https://www.hopkinsmedicine.org/health/conditions-and-diseases/constipation-causes-and-prevention-tips. Accessed December 20, 2020.
[3] Dobarrio-Sanz I, Hernandez-Padilla JM, Lopez-Rodriguez MM, et al. Non-pharmacological interventions to improve constipation amongst older adults in long-term care settings: a systematic review of randomized controlled trials. Geriatr Nurs 2020;7(12):992–9.
[4] The Lancet. The cost of constipation. Lancet Gastroenterol Hepato 2019;4:811.
[5] Warraich HJ. First opinion. Beyond aggravation: constipation is an American epidemic. STAT News 2017. Available at: https://www.statnews.com/2017/08/17/constipation-bowels-colon/. Accessed December 20, 2020.
[6] De Giorgio R, Ruggeri E, Stanghellini V, et al. Chronic constipation in the elderly: a primer for the gastroenterologist. BMC Gastroenterol 2015;15(130):1–13, 130-143.

[7] Centers for Medicare & Medicaid Services. National health expenditure fact sheet. 2020. Available at: https://www.cms.gov/Research-Statistics-Data-and-Systems/Statistics-Trends-and-Reports/NationalHealthExpendData/NHE-Fact-Sheet. Accessed December 20, 2020.

[8] Andrews CN, Storr M. The pathophysiology of chronic constipation. Can J Gastroenterol 2011;25(Suppl B):16B–21B.

[9] Cleveland Clinic. Pelvic floor dysfunction: diagnosis and tests. 2020. https://my.cleveland-clinic.org/health/diseases/14459-pelvic-floor-dysfunction/diagnosis-and-tests. Accessed December 20, 2020.

[10] Rome Foundation. Understanding functional gastrointestinal disorders. 2016. Available at: https://theromefoundation.org/rome-iv/whats-new-for-rome-iv/. Accessed December 20, 2020.

[11] Schmulson MJ, Drossman DA. What is new inn Rome IV. J Neurogastroenterol Motil 2017;23(2):151–63.

[12] Aziz I, Whitehead WD, Palsson OS, et al. An approach to the diagnosis and management of Rome IV functional disorders of chronic constipation. Expert Rev Gastroenterol Hepatol 2020;14(1):39–46.

[13] Palsson OS, Whitehead W, Tornblom H, et al. Prevalence of Rome IV functional bowel disorders among adults in the United States, Canada, and the United Kingdom. Gastroenterol 2020;158:1262–73.

[14] Lacy BE, Patel NK. Rome criteria and a diagnostic approach to irritable bowel syndrome. J Clin Med 2017;6(11):99–106.

[15] Drossman DA. Functional gastrointestinal disorders: history, pathophysiology, clinical features, and Rome IV. Gastroenterol 2016;150:1262–79.

[16] Thomas-Henkel C, Schulman M. Screening for social determinants of health in populations with complex needs: implementation considerations. Center for Health Care Strategies, Inc.; 2017. Available at: http://www.chcs.org/media/SDOH-Complex-Care-Screening-Brief-102617.pdf. Accessed December 20, 2020.

[17] Centers for Disease Control and Prevention. Social determinants of health 2020. Available at: https://www.cdc.gov/publichealthgateway/sdoh/index.html. Accessed December 20, 2020.

[18] Centers for Disease Control and Prevention. About social determinants of health 2020. Available at: https://www.cdc.gov/socialdeterminants/about.html. Accessed December 20, 2020.

[19] Rekstis E. Poop and you. Healthline 2019. Available at: https://www.healthline.com/health/digestive-health/types-of-poop. Accessed December 21, 2020.

[20] Fortin AH VI. Chapter 32. Constipation. IN: Henderson MC, Tierney LM, Smetana GW. eds The Patient History: An evidence-based approach to differential diagnosis. McGraw-Hill. Available at: https://accessmedicine.mhmedical.com/content.aspx?bookid=500&sectionid=41026580. Accessed December 21, 2020.

[21] Rao SSC, Meduri K. What is necessary to diagnose constipation? Best Pract Res Clin Gastroenterol 2011;25(1):127–40.

[22] Paquette IM, Varma M, Ternent C, et al. The American Society of Colon and Rectal Surgeon's clinical practice guideline for the evaluation and management of constipation. Dis Colon Rectum 2016;59:479–92.

[23] Hayat U, Dugum M, Garg S. Chronic constipation: update on management. Cleve Clin J Med 2017;84(5):397–408.

[24] Mearin F, Ciriza C, Mínguez M, et al. Clinical practice guideline: irritable bowel syndrome with constipation and functional constipation in the adult. Rev Esp Enferm Dig 2016;108:332–63.

[25] Sobrado CW, Corrêa Neto IJF, Pinto RA, et al. Diagnosis and treatment of constipation: a clinical update based on the Rome IV criteria. J Coloproctoly (Rio de Janeiro) 2018;38(2):137–44.

[26] Bharucha AE, Wald A. Chronic constipation. Mayo Clin Proc 2019;94(11):2340–57.

Diagnosis and Management of Dementia in Primary Care

Elizabeth Galik, PhD, CRNP

University of Maryland School of Nursing, 655 West Lombard Street, 375C, Baltimore, MD 21201, USA

Keywords

- Dementia • Alzheimer disease • Mental status examination • Cognition
- Neurocognitive disorder • Delirium

Key points

- Primary care providers are in a unique position to utilize case finding approaches for patients who do have cognitive symptoms that could be due to dementia.
- The differential diagnosis of dementia includes delirium, depression, age-related memory impairment, and minor cognitive impairment.
- The mental status examination is a critical component of the patient assessment when dementia, delirium, or psychiatric syndromes are suspected.
- The presence and active involvement of a caregiver are fundamental components of longitudinal care for individuals living with dementia.
- The use of psychotropic medications, such as antipsychotics, antidepressants, mood stabilizers, and benzodiazepines, should be minimized among individuals living with dementia unless the behavioral symptoms are severe and the potential benefits of the medication outweigh the potential risks.

INTRODUCTION

Dementia is a term used to describe the presence of a major neurocognitive disorder that results in impairment in memory, language, problem-solving ability, executive dysfunction, and/or other symptoms that are severe enough to cause changes in an individual's ability to function [1]. Although there are many different disorders that result in dementia, Alzheimer disease is the most

The author has no financial conflicts of interest.

E-mail address: galik@umaryland.edu

https://doi.org/10.1016/j.yfpn.2021.01.001
2589-420X/21/© 2021 Elsevier Inc. All rights reserved.

prevalent cause and accounts for 60% to 80% of all individuals with dementia [2]. It is estimated that there are 5 million to 6 million individuals in the United States who are living with Alzheimer disease, and the cost to the nation is more than $305 billion [2]. In part due to an aging population, the prevalence of persons living with dementia is increasing; however, it is under-recognized and many individuals are not diagnosed until later stages of the disease. Although the US Preventative Services Task Force has concluded that there is insufficient evidence to support cognitive screening for asymptomatic older adults, primary care providers are in a unique position to utilize case finding approaches for patients who do have cognitive symptoms that could be due to dementia. The annual Medicare wellness visit provides an excellent opportunity for case finding. The purpose of this article is to describe the assessment, differential diagnosis, and management of dementia.

DEMENTIA HISTORY

Although Alzheimer disease is the most common cause of dementia, there are several other causes of dementia, including cerebrovascular disease (vascular dementia), Lewy body dementia, frontotemporal dementia, Parkinson disease dementia, mixed dementia, and others. Defining history characteristics of each type of dementia are described in Table 1. Despite these differences, early symptoms and traits can overlap and in late stages of dementia, it may be difficult to distinguish these different subtypes. When obtaining a history, it is important to elicit the chief complaint from the patient because this helps to assess his/her insight into any symptoms or deficits. Meeting with the patient first helps to build trust between the patient and provider and allows for the patient to communicate any concerns and describe symptoms and perceptions without relying on other informants. In many cases, the patient may lack insight into cognitive, functional, and behavioral symptoms, but it remains important to listen to the patient's perceptions.

The history of the present illness should be described and verified by 1 or more reliable informants when evaluating a patient for possible dementia. Informants, such as family members, friends, coworkers, other health care providers, and neighbors, may accompany the patient to the initial visit, or the health care provider may need to gain the patient's permission to contact a reliable informant by telephone. The informant should be asked about the onset and course of changes in cognition, function, and behavior and the manner of symptom progression, as highlighted in Table 1. The AD8 is a brief informant survey instrument with established validity and reliability that can be used to collect relevant history about symptoms that are consistent with dementia [3,4].

Family history should focus on the history of dementia, psychiatric disorders, and neurologic conditions of grandparents, parents, siblings, and children, if known. Age and cause of death also can be helpful information to determine if family members lived to an age of risk for dementia or died earlier due to another cause. Family member response and tolerance to pharmacologic

Table 1
Defining history characteristics for different types of dementia

Type of dementia	Onset and course	Cognition	Function	Behavior
Alzheimer disease	Insidious onset and gradually progressive	Gradual decline over time in memory, language, and perceptual recognition; decreased insight into cognitive deficits	Gradual decline over time with accompanying motor apraxia	Depression, psychotic symptoms, and sundowning symptoms are common.
Vascular dementia	More likely to be sudden with stepwise progression	More likely to be sudden with stepwise progression; challenges with executive functioning; tend to have some insight into deficits early in the dementia	Varies depending on location of cerebrovascular damage	Varies depending on location of cerebrovascular damage
Lewy body dementia	Gradual and progressive with cognitive, motor, and psychotic symptoms occurring together and early in the disease process	Gradual and progressive, often with significant decline in language ability	Parkinsonism is common early in the disease process and has a negative impact on function.	Psychosis is common early in the disease; prominent visual hallucinations typically at night.
Frontotemporal dementia	Gradual and progressive	Decreased insight with impulsivity; May have an impact on language	Lack of safety awareness has a negative impact on functional ability.	Personality changes, impulsive, disinhibited behaviors are common.
Parkinson disease dementia	Gradual and progressive	Decline is gradual and occurs approximately 5–7 y after the onset of motor symptoms; executive dysfunction is prominent early.	Decline in function is negatively impacted by motor and cognitive symptoms.	Depression and psychotic symptoms are common.

treatments for psychiatric disorders also may be warranted if the patient is experiencing a neuropsychiatric complication associated with dementia.

Personal history includes educational attainment, occupation, hobbies/interests, sources of social support, premorbid personality, and current living arrangements. If there has been a change in living arrangements, perhaps from the patient's home to an adult child's home, it is helpful to determine the symptoms that precipitated the move. Current and past tobacco, alcohol, and substance use also should be assessed, ideally with a reliable and valid screening instrument.

The patient's medical history should include a summary of comorbid medical conditions with year of diagnosis if known, surgical history, and a complete list of medications and supplements with dose and frequency. Particular attention should be paid to medications that can have a negative impact on cognition, such as anticholinergic medications, such as diphenhydramine, narcotics, antipsychotics, benzodiazepines, sedative/hypnotics, mood stabilizers/anticonvulsants, and antidepressants. A complete review of systems also is important to gather because it can help identify additional symptoms that may be related to an unstable medical condition, adverse medication side effect, or acute delirium. Any recent falls, trauma, or safety concerns also should be elucidated and a thorough review of systems should be completed.

DEMENTIA ASSESSMENT

The physical examination of the patient with suspected dementia should be confirmatory with the patient's history and generally includes a complete cardiovascular, peripheral vascular, neurologic, and musculoskeletal examination. Additional examination components may be necessary to rule out potential causes of delirium. Assessment of the patient's gait balance, muscle strength, and reflexes should be conducted, and any extrapyramidal symptoms, such as tremor, drooling, increased tone, cogwheeling, and dyskinesia, should be noted. A patient with early Alzheimer disease is likely to have a normal physical examination; however, those with moderate to severe Alzheimer disease may exhibit gait changes, increasing motor apraxia, and increased peripheral tone. Those with Alzheimer disease and at the end of life may exhibit primitive reflexes, also called frontal release signs, such as the suck, snout, palmomental, and grasp reflexes [5]. A patient with vascular dementia is more likely to have cardiovascular abnormalities, such as carotid bruit, atrial fibrillation, and peripheral arterial disease; gait changes; and a focal neurologic examination (facial droop, dysarthria, hyperreflexia, and decreased strength); however, these findings may not always be diagnostic. Examination findings consistent with parkinsonism are associated more commonly with Lewy body dementia and Parkinson disease dementia but also may result from the use of antipsychotic medications, metoclopramide, and/or prochlorperazine.

The mental status examination also is a critical component of the patient assessment when dementia, delirium, or other psychiatric syndromes are suspected. Several factors, such as educational level, primary language, sensory deficits, and impaired baseline intellectual function, may influence a patient's performance on the mental status examination, in particular, assessment of cognition. The mental status examination is composed of an assessment of level of consciousness, appearance and behavior, speech and language, mood, thought process and content, and cognition. Brief cognitive screening instruments, such as the Mini-Mental State Examination [6], Mini-Cog [7], and the Montreal Cognitive Assessment [8] can be used to objectively screen for cognitive impairment. Table 2 provides an overview of the components of the mental status examination and describes ways to assess each component.

PATHOPHYSIOLOGY

The pathophysiology of dementia varies widely depending on the cause or type of disorder, and the exact pathophysiologic mechanisms are poorly understood for several types of dementia. Alzheimer disease, the most common cause of dementia, has been associated with the presence of β-amyloid protein deposits on neurons and tau neurofibrillary tangles within neurons. In addition to the presence of these abnormal proteins, there are disruptions to neurotransmitters, such as acetylcholine and serotonin, chronic inflammation, disruptions in glucose metabolism, and changes in cerebral blood flow. Some of these changes may be present in a preclinical phase of Alzheimer disease that is estimated to occur at least 10 years prior to the onset of clinical symptoms of Alzheimer disease.

As Alzheimer disease progresses, there is continued neuronal cell death with resulting severe cortical atrophy. The neuronal atrophy associated with Alzheimer disease is most common in the frontal and temporal lobes and the

Table 2	
Components of the mental status examination	
Component	**Considerations for assessment**
Level of consciousness	Awake and alert, lethargic, fluctuating, or hypervigilant; level of attention and eye contact; Richmond Agitation-Sedation Scale [18]
Appearance and behavior	Dress, grooming, motor behavior
Speech and language	Spontaneous speech; hesitation; delay; word finding difficulty; paraphasias; rate, rhythm, and volume
Mood	Mood, anhedonia, vital sense, feelings of guilt or self-deprecation, outlook on the future; Cornell Scale for Depression in Dementia [19]
Thought content and process	Delusions, hallucinations, bizarre thoughts
Insight and judgment	The patient's awareness of self and condition; ability to identify behavior that may be harmful
Cognition	Orientation, short-term and long-term memory, verbal fluency, executive functioning; Mini-Mental State Examination [6]; Mini-Cog [7]; Montreal Cognitive Assessment [8]

ventricles frequently are enlarged as the dementia syndrome progresses. Unfortunately, the presence of ventricular enlargement and cortical atrophy in Alzheimer disease is a nonspecific and also may be seen in the normal aging brain. Additionally, there are genetic mutations that appear to increase the risk of developing Alzheimer disease. The Alzheimer's Disease Education and Referral Center, sponsored by the National Institute on Aging, provides an educational video that can be used for provider and patient education and is available at https://www.nia.nih.gov/health/video-how-alzheimers-changes-brain?
utm_source=ADvideo&utm_medium=web&utm_campaign=rightrail.

DIFFERENTIAL DIAGNOSIS

According to the *Diagnostic and Statistical Manual of Mental Disorders* (Fifth Edition) (*DSM-5*), in order to diagnose dementia, otherwise known as neurocognitive disorder, the patient must meet the following diagnostic criteria [1].

- Significant cognitive decline must be present from baseline in 1 or more of the following areas: memory, perception, motor ability, attention, or executive function
- The cognitive impairments result in some dependence in day-to-day activities, such as managing finances, administering medications, cooking, arranging transportation, grooming, dressing. and other activities of daily living.
- These cognitive deficits occur in the absence of delirium.
- The cognitive deficits are not better associated with or explained by a psychiatric disorder, such as depression or schizophrenia.

Unlike dementia, when changes in cognition, function, and behavior occur insidiously, delirium is a disorder that results in an acute change in mental status. According to the *DSM-5*, delirium is a disorder that has an impact on attention and awareness that develops suddenly and is fluctuating in nature [1]. Delirium has direct physiologic consequences and is caused by a medical condition, intoxication of a substance, an adverse reaction to medication, or multiple causes. Delirium commonly is associated with negative health outcomes, such as cognitive decline, functional decline, long-term care placement, and death. Like dementia, delirium is under-recognized and is diagnosed in only half of individuals who display symptoms. The fluctuating level of alertness, attention, confusion, and misperceptions of reality that commonly are seen in delirium also are noted among other disorders, such as dementia, acute psychiatric disorders, and depression. Additionally, delirium can co-occur with these other disorders, which make differential diagnosis even more challenging. Lastly, dementia is perhaps the most significant risk factor for developing delirium, and episodes of delirium can hasten the cognitive, functional, and behavioral decline often seen in dementia. This bidirectional relationship between dementia and delirium further complicates assessment, diagnosis, and treatment. Some widely used valid and reliable screening tools for delirium include the Confusion Assessment Method [9], which is based on patient observation, and the Delirium Rating Scale [10], which utilizes an informant report. Table 3 provides a comparison of the characteristics of dementia, delirium, and depression that can be utilized for differential diagnosis. In some instances, depression can mimic the presentation of dementia and include symptoms, such as difficulty making decisions, forgetfulness, apathy, and psychomotor retardation, coupled with depressed mood and/or anhedonia.

Dementia also should be distinguished from individuals with age-related memory impairment and mild cognitive impairment (MCI). The primary symptom associated with age-related subjective memory impairment, sometimes called normal cognitive aging, includes a slowed processing speed. Other symptoms can include occasional difficulty but not inability to access names and the requirement for additional time to learn new things. These symptoms are not associated with any decline in daily function and the individual is able to live independently and objective cognitive testing is normal. MCI is a disorder that results in a measurable mild impairment in 1 or more cognitive domains (typically memory is involved) but is not severe enough to cause impairment in activities of daily living. Typically, neuropsychological testing battery is required to support a diagnosis of MCI. Approximately 50% of individuals with MCI go on to develop a progressive dementia disorder, such as Alzheimer disease or vascular dementia; however, currently, there is no way to predict which individuals will progress to dementia.

DIAGNOSTIC TESTING
- Diagnostic tests essentially rule out potentially treatable conditions because there are no diagnostic tests to definitively diagnose dementia.
- The cause of dementia is based on a clinical diagnosis, so symptom description and progression are important whereas examination findings and results from diagnostic testing tend to be confirmatory.
- The type of dementia can be diagnosed definitively only after death following a brain autopsy.
- Laboratory studies that typically are ordered to rule out various metabolic conditions: comprehensive metabolic panel, complete blood cell count, thyroid-stimulating hormone, vitamin B_{12}, and folate

Table 3
Comparison of characteristics associated with dementia, delirium, and depression

Characteristic	Dementia	Delirium	Depression
Onset	Gradual	Sudden	Gradual
Course	Insidious	Fluctuates	Gradual
Attention	Intact	Disrupted, distractible	Intact, but slowed
Lethargy	Uncommon but apathy is possible	Fluctuating level of consciousness	Common
Psychosis	Possible, typically in moderate stages	Hallucinations are more common	Possible, typically with severe depression, mood congruent

- Depending on a patient's history and risk factors, the health care provider also may consider ordering rapid plasma reagin, human immunodeficiency virus screen, toxicology screen, sedimentation rate/carcinoembryonic antigen for inflammation, and/or urinalysis and culture.
- Brain imaging (computed tomography or magnetic resonance imaging) may be ordered to rule out a stroke, tumor, or bleed. An single-photon emission computed tomography scan that shows significant decreased blood flow to the frontal and temporal lobe may be suggestive of frontotemporal dementia.
- A carotid ultrasound may be warranted if there is clear history of ischemic stroke(s).

DEMENTIA MANAGEMENT

Treatment of the patient living with dementia includes (1) supportive care of the patient, (2) addressing caregiver needs, and (3) consideration of possible pharmacologic interventions to treat cognitive symptoms associated with dementia.

Supportive care of the patient includes interventions designed to promote quality of life, safety, and fulfillment of the patient's wishes throughout the course of the disorder. These supportive interventions often are achieved in conjunction with caregivers and include but are not limited to the following:

- Legal protection: obtaining durable medical and financial power of attorney and advanced directives while the patient is still able to participate in decision making
- Safety: addressing common safety concerns, such as motor vehicle accidents, wandering, elopement, accidents in the home, lack of medication adherence, and so forth. The patient may benefit from a functional driving evaluation, assistance with medication administration, a home safety evaluation, environmental modifications, or some level of increased monitoring, supervision, or assistance.
- Emphasizing structure and a daily routine with opportunities for the patient to participate in meaningful activities
- Assuring adequate nutrition, hydration, and physical activity
- Prevention of acute illnesses and stability of chronic illness through recommended immunizations, physical activity, and regular medical appointments to address medical comorbidities

The presence and active involvement of a caregiver are fundamental components of longitudinal care for individuals living with dementia. In addition to addressing the needs of the patient living with dementia, it also is important to meet the needs of the caregiver. Suggestions include

- Education about dementia symptoms, progression, and anticipatory guidance: helpful resources are available from the National Institute on Aging, https://www.nia.nih.gov/health/topics/dementia, and the Alzheimer's Association, https://www.alz.org/.
- Referral to community resources: in-home services, senior centers, day program, respite services, and support groups
- Comfort and emotional support
- Teaching the caregiver strategies to manage behavioral symptoms of distress and optimize function and physical activity. Some helpful educational/training

videos include caregiver training videos produced by the University of California, Los Angeles, https://www.uclahealth.org/dementia/caregiver-education-videos, and the Function Focused Care training videos https://functionfocusedcare.wordpress.com/video-coaching/.

Pharmacologic interventions to treat the cognitive symptoms of Alzheimer disease include cholinesterase inhibitors (donepezil, rivastigmine, and galantamine) and the N-methyl D-aspartate, memantine. Cholinesterase inhibitors may temporarily provide some stabilization or slight improvement in cognition or function among individuals living with Alzheimer disease [11,12]. Rivastigmine is the only cholinesterase inhibitor to have an indication for the treatment of Parkinson disease dementia. Table 4 provides an overview of prescribing guidelines for cholinesterase inhibitors. Common adverse effects from cholinesterase inhibitors include gastrointestinal upset, bradycardia, syncope, and nightmares/vivid dreams. Guidelines for the discontinuation of cholinesterase inhibitors can be found in a recent article in the *American Journal of Geriatric Psychiatry*, https://pubmed.ncbi.nlm.nih.gov/29167065/ [13].

Almost all individuals with dementia experience behavioral symptoms of distress or neuropsychiatric symptoms at some point during the course of their illness. Behavioral symptoms of distress include symptoms, such as motor restlessness, wandering, resistiveness to care, verbal and/or physical aggression, repetitive vocalizations, mood disturbances, psychotic symptoms, and sleep disturbances. Although behavioral symptoms of distress frequently are time

Table 4
Cholinesterase prescribing guidelines (for patients without hepatic and renal impairment)

Donepezil	• 5–10 mg qd (mild to moderate Alzheimer disease) • 23 mg (moderate to severe Alzheimer disease)	• 5 mg qd 4–6 wk, then 10 mg as tolerated • 10 mg qd for 3 mo before considering increase to 23 mg
Galantamine	• 8–16 mg bid • 8 mg ER–16 mg ER • 24 mg ER/day	• 4 mg bid 4–6 wk, then 8 mg bid 4–6 wk, then 12 mg bid • 8 mg ER–16 mg ER if tolerated after 4 wk; May increase to 24 mg ER/day after 4 weeks if tolerated
Rivastigmine (also indicated for Parkinson disease dementia)	• 3–6 mg bid • 4.6 mg–9.5 mg patch	• Oral dosing: 1.5 mg bid for 2–4 wk, 3 mg bid for 2–4 wk, then 4.5 mg bid for 2–4 wk, then 6 mg bid • Transdermal patch: 4.6 mg/24 h once a day for 4 wk then increase to 9.5 mg/24 h once a day if tolerated to reach first treatment dose; Further titration to 13.3 mg/24 h once a day may be warranted

Abbreviation: ER, extended release

limited, there are no medications approved by the Food and Drug Administration to treat these symptoms. Nonpharmacologic interventions, such as sensory stimulation activities (music, massage, and touch), cognitive stimulation activities, emotion-oriented interventions (reminiscence, validation, and simulated presence), physical activity and exercise, and behavioral education and training for caregivers should be used as first-line treatment in the management of behavioral symptoms in the context of dementia. Pharmacologic management of behavioral symptoms, in particular, the use of antipsychotics, among individuals living with dementia has limited effectiveness and is associated with significant risks, such as, sedation, falls, fractures, delirium, motor symptoms, cardiovascular complications, stroke, pneumonia, and death [14–17]. The use of psychotropic medications, such as antipsychotics, antidepressants, mood stabilizers, and benzodiazepines, should be minimized among individuals living with dementia unless the behavioral symptoms are severe and the potential benefits of the medication outweigh the potential risks.

SUMMARY

- Most primary care providers can diagnose and manage most patients with dementia successfully; however, in some cases, when symptom presentation is atypical, neuropsychiatric symptoms are severe and unresponsive to treatment, and the age of onset of cognitive impairment begins before age 60, then referral to a cognitive neurologist, geriatric specialist, or geriatric psychiatric provider may be warranted.
- Ideally, team-based care that includes nurses, physicians, social workers, pharmacists, and rehabilitation therapists can work together to support the health and well-being of the patient and caregiver dyad.

CLINICS CARE POINTS

- Almost all individuals with dementia experience behavioral symptoms of distress or neuropsychiatric symptoms at some point during the course of their illness. Anticipatory guidance regarding the likelihood of behavioral symptoms of distress is important for early identification and treatment.
- Delirium superimposed on dementia leads to more rapid cognitive, functional and behavioral decline and delirium screening is important if there is a sudden change in the patient's condition.

References
[1] American Psychiatric Association. Diagnostic and statistical manual of mental disorders (DSM-5). 5th edition. Washington, DC: American Psychiatric Publishing; 2013.
[2] Alzheimer's Association. 2020 Alzheimer's disease facts and figures. 2020. Available at: https://www.alz.org/media/Documents/alzheimers-facts-and-figures.pdf. Accessed August 24, 2020.
[3] Galvin JE, Roe CM, Powlishta KK, et al. The AD8: a brief informant interview to detect dementia. Neurology 2005;65(4):559–64.
[4] Galvin JE, Roe CM, Xiong C, et al. Validity and reliability of the AD8 informant interview in dementia. Neurology 2006;67(11):1942–8.
[5] Walker HK. The suck, snout, palmomental, and grasp reflexes. In: Walker HK, Hall WD, Hurst JW, editors. Clinical methods: the history, physical, and laboratory examinations.

3rd edition. Chapter 71, 363-364. Boston: Butterworths; 1990. Available at: http://www.ncbi.nlm.nih.gov/books/NBK395/. Accessed August 29, 2020.

[6] Folstein MF, Folstein SE, McHugh PR. "Mini-mental state". A practical method for grading the cognitive state of patients for the clinician. J Psychiatr Res 1975;12(3):189–98.

[7] Borson S, Scanlan JM, Chen P, et al. The Mini-Cog as a screen for dementia: validation in a population-based sample. J Am Geriatr Soc 2003;51(10):1451–4.

[8] Nasreddine ZS, Phillips NA, Bédirian V, et al. The Montreal Cognitive Assessment, MoCA: a brief screening tool for mild cognitive impairment. J Am Geriatr Soc 2005;53(4):695–9.

[9] Inouye SK, van Dyck CH, Alessi CA, et al. Clarifying confusion: the confusion assessment method. A new method for detection of delirium. Ann Intern Med 1990;113(12):941–8.

[10] Trzepacz PT, Baker RW, Greenhouse J. A symptom rating scale for delirium. Psychiatry Res 1988;23(1):89–97.

[11] Birks J. Cholinesterase inhibitors for Alzheimer's disease. Cochrane Database Syst Rev 2006;(1):CD005593.

[12] Knight R, Khondoker M, Magill N, et al. A systematic review and meta-analysis of the effectiveness of acetylcholinesterase inhibitors and memantine in treating the cognitive symptoms of dementia. Dement Geriatr Cogn Disord 2018;45(3–4):131–51.

[13] Renn BN, Asghar-Ali AA, Thielke S, et al. A systematic review of practice guidelines and recommendations for discontinuation of cholinesterase inhibitors in dementia. Am J Geriatr Psychiatry 2018;26(2):134–47.

[14] Corbett A, Ballard C. Antipsychotics and mortality in dementia. Am J Psychiatry 2012;169(1):7–9.

[15] Brännström J, Boström G, Rosendahl E, et al. Psychotropic drug use and mortality in old people with dementia: investigating sex differences. BMC Pharmacol Toxicol 2017;18(1):36.

[16] Galik E, Resnick B. Psychotropic medication use and association with physical and psychosocial outcomes in nursing home residents. J Psychiatr Ment Health Nurs 2012; https://doi.org/10.1111/j.1365-2850.2012.01911.x.

[17] Maust DT, Langa KM, Blow FC, et al. Psychotropic use and associated neuropsychiatric symptoms among patients with dementia in the USA. Int J Geriatr Psychiatry 2017;32(2):164–74.

[18] Sessler CN, Gosnell MS, Grap MJ, et al. The Richmond Agitation-Sedation Scale: validity and reliability in adult intensive care unit patients. Am J Respir Crit Care Med 2002;166(10):1338–44.

[19] Alexopoulos GS, Abrams RC, Young RC, et al. Cornell scale for depression in dementia. Biol Psychiatry 1988;23(3):271–84.

Women's Health

Evidence-Based Care for Pregnancy Complicated by Obesity
What Primary Care Providers Should Know

Elizabeth Muñoz, MSN, CNM*, Ellen Solis, DNP, CNM,
Vanessa Grafton, MSN, CNM

Carle Foundation Hospital, 611 West Park Street, Urbana, IL 61801, USA

Keywords
• Pregnancy • Obesity • Bias • Family nurse practitioner • Prenatal care

Key points

- Family nurse practitioners should know the current recommendations of care for pregnant people with body mass index (BMI) greater than 40 $kg.m^2$ and be able to refer to an appropriate pregnancy provider.
- Initiating prenatal care in the first trimester is a key component for a healthy pregnancy and aids in the identification of risk factors, including obesity, hypertension, and glucose intolerance.
- It is important for family nurse practitioners to assess their biases regarding pregnant people with obesity and focus on inclusive changes to their practices, such as incorporating people-first language.
- All patients should be informed of their risks in pregnancy, including those with a BMI greater than 40.0 kg/m^2.
- A checklist is a helpful tool for nurse practitioners to use when caring for pregnant patients with BMI more than 40.0 kg/m^2.

INTRODUCTION

Obesity in pregnancy is a common occurrence in the United States and the obesity rate continues to increase annually [1–4]. Having obesity during pregnancy increases the risk of complications and poor outcomes for both the pregnant person and fetus [2]. As the incidence of obesity in pregnancy

*Corresponding author. E-mail address: elizabethgmunoz@gmail.com

https://doi.org/10.1016/j.yfpn.2021.01.008
2589-420X/21/© 2021 Elsevier Inc. All rights reserved.

and associated comorbidities increase, family nurse practitioners (FNPs) frequently encounter these patients and should familiarize themselves with some specific points when caring for pregnant people with obesity. This article explores what FNPs should know to initiate care for pregnant patients with obesity, including components of the first prenatal appointment, options for the patient to receive an appropriate referral for prenatal care, and a review of the latest evidence for this patient population. Providers can reference Appendix A for an evidence-based guide when caring for this patient population.

Significance

According to the Pregnancy Risk Assessment Monitoring System (PRAMS), 25.3% of women in the United States are obese before conceiving a pregnancy [5]. The obesity problem in America continues to grow and increases the risks of other health complications, such as hypertension, other cardiovascular diseases, and diabetes [6]. These increased risk factors can be present when a patient with obesity is pregnant and can occur at any point in the pregnancy [7,8].

An increase in obstetric complications can negatively affect the life of the patient during the pregnancy, such as with additional appointments needed for care. In contrast, going without the recommended interventions can lead to negative pregnancy outcomes for both the patient and fetus. Table 1 provides a concise list of evidence-based steps for FNPs to follow when establishing prenatal care for a patient with obesity. By understanding the risks of pregnancy complicated by obesity, FNPs can provide care that can lead to better pregnancy outcomes, is in line with the latest evidence, and can mitigate risk for this patient population.

Assessment

Diagnosis. Obesity is defined by the Centers for Disease Control and Prevention (CDC) as a BMI greater than 30.0 kg/m^2 [9–11]. The prevalence of obesity continues to increase in the United States, including in pregnant people [5]. Obesity is a condition with causes that are multifactorial and include increased exposure to stressors, caloric intake and energy output, and genetics [9]. The diagnosis of obesity is associated with an increase of other comorbidities, such as diabetes mellitus and cardiovascular disease, as well as depression and anxiety. For these reasons, it is important to screen for obesity early in

Table 1
Definitions and classes of obesity

Obesity is defined as BMI $\geq$30.0 kg/m^2	Class 1 obesity is a BMI of 30.0–34.9 kg/m^2
The measurement of BMI is taken at the first prenatal visit	Class 2 obesity is 35.0–39.9 kg/m^2
	Class 3 obesity is 40.0 kg/m^2 or higher
Use the patient's prepregnant weight to calculate BMI	

pregnancy to ensure that any comorbidities are identified and addressed for the pregnant patient. Table 1 summarizes key points about screening for obesity in pregnancy and further breaks down the 3 classes of obesity.

Preconception visit. Ideally, anyone planning pregnancy should have a preconception discussion with a provider well before pregnancy. Although this visit does not always occur as a formal preconception visit, if the provider has the opportunity to counsel the patient on healthy choices (weight control, immunizations, smoking, and substance use, and so forth) before pregnancy is achieved, there is potential that pregnancy complications could be avoided. Research also shows that those affected by obesity are particularly vulnerable to pregnancy-related complications and are therefore more likely to benefit from professional advice and counseling [12]. This discussion can also take place at an annual examination or problem-focused visits where the provider can take the opportunity to offer preconception counseling (or contraception if pregnancy is not desired) outside of a formal preconception visit.

Perhaps most beneficially, a preconception discussion allows a discussion of the potential risks of infertility and spontaneous abortion and for specific advice on the benefits of weight loss before conception. Multiple studies have shown an increase in the risk of spontaneous abortion in patients with a BMI more than 25 kg/m^2 compared with those with a BMI less than 25 kg/m^2 [13]. These risks are hypothesized to be associated with hormonal alterations and endometrial receptivity in patients with an increased BMI [14]. Clients with obesity who have experienced multiple spontaneous abortions or who are experiencing infertility may benefit from a referral to an infertility specialist [14].

A prepregnancy reduction in BMI is one of the most effective ways of mitigating risk and seems to have an overall positive effect on reproductive function. Schummers and colleagues [15] found that a 10% reduction in prepregnancy BMI could reduce the risk of preeclampsia, gestational diabetes, macrosomia, stillbirth, and indicated preterm birth by 10%. In addition to this, these researchers found that a 20% to 30% weight loss could reduce the risks of cesarean section and shoulder dystocia [15]. Effective counseling on diet, exercise, and behavior modification should be provided, along with the possibility of medical therapies or bariatric surgery. This counseling can be given through providing information on the effects of obesity in pregnancy along with specific advice on healthy food choices and exercise. The involvement of dieticians, exercise experts, and bariatric specialists may also help clients to achieve these weight loss goals [16].

Initial prenatal visit. Although a preconception visit is an opportunity to discuss the known antepartum complications of obesity in pregnancy and promote healthy habits, a client may not present to care until pregnancy is achieved. It is therefore crucial to document a careful medical, surgical, and family history and address the known complications of obesity at an initial prenatal visit. The details of prenatal care vary from practice to practice, but the goal is always to initiate care early and to ensure health for the pregnant person and fetus. The critical components of prenatal care include:

- Early and accurate establishment of gestational age
- Identification of risk factors that could increase morbidity and mortality
- Measurement of weight and calculation of BMI
- Comprehensive and ongoing assessment of maternal and fetal health
- Anticipation of problems that might occur during pregnancy
- Counseling on ways to avoid identified health problems
- Shared decision making, education, health promotion, and support throughout pregnancy

Understanding the pregnant person's health history enables the provider to order appropriate laboratory evaluation, provide guidance on available genetic testing, and support the health of the pregnancy.

The pregnant person's medical history guides decisions about laboratory tests, genetic screenings, and diagnostic tests, and can begin with details of the current pregnancy. Accurate dating of the pregnancy is crucial in managing the pregnancy, offering genetic screenings, and monitoring fetal growth. Several calculators are available to help establish the estimated date of delivery (EDD) based on the last menstrual period (LMP) using Naegele's rule. See Table 2 for a Naegele's rule calculator. If the client's menses are irregular or the LMP is not known, ultrasonography examination of the fetus before 20 weeks' gestation can provide a reliable estimation of fetal size and the EDD. Many providers prefer ultrasonography estimation of the EDD for all pregnancies; however, the client's preference and financial constraints could make this difficult, and an accurate LMP is always desirable.

The medical history should also include risk factors for ectopic pregnancy (history of pelvic infection or previous ectopic pregnancy), menstrual history (age of menarche and regularity of menses), cardiac disease, hypertension, diabetes, chronic medical conditions such as asthma, lung disease, frequent urinary tract infections, allergies, immunization history, dietary restrictions (such as a history of phenylketonuria), history or risk for sexually transmitted infections, travel, and any other factors that could affect the pregnant person's health. The medical history should also include a review of the client's past obstetric history, with special attention to a history of frequent miscarriage, still

Table 2
Naegele's rule

Naegele's rule: LMP + 9 mo + add 7 d		
Step 1	Use first day of last menstrual period	December 15, 2020
Step 2	Add 9 mo	September 15
Step 3	Add 7 d	September 22, 2021

birth, preeclampsia, gestational diabetes, preterm labor and birth, fetal anomalies, shoulder dystocia, postpartum hemorrhage, and any other complications of pregnancy or birth.

A comprehensive surgical history should include any uterine surgeries (cesarean section, myomectomy, and laparoscopic surgery), reasons for surgeries, and reaction to anesthesia. If the client has undergone a cesarean section in the past, it is important to provide counseling and develop a plan for a trial of labor after cesarean or a repeat cesarean.

Understanding the client's family history is also important in supporting a healthy pregnancy. A family history of heritable disorders that could affect the fetus, genetic diseases (known or suspected), fetal malformations, intellectual disability, autism spectrum disorders, and consanguinity should all be documented, and appropriate counseling and testing offered [17]. Electronic medical record systems designed for documentation of pregnancy provide easy-to-use guides for documenting all aspects of the client's medical, surgical, and obstetric history.

Another important component of the initial prenatal visit is a comprehensive psychosocial history. Psychosocial issues that should be discussed include whether the pregnancy was planned or unintended, potential barriers to care (such as transportation problems, language barriers, work schedules, economic constraints, and childcare), housing concerns, intimate partner violence, substance use, and mental health. Identifying these concerns can help the provider make suggestions and appropriate referrals early in the pregnancy and to follow up on any identified issues as pregnancy progresses. Validated mental health screening tools such as the Edinburgh Postnatal Depression Scale the Patient Healthcare Questionnaire-2, or Patient Healthcare Questionnaire-9 should be used at least once in every pregnancy to help identify mental health disorders that can affect the client's pregnancy and ability to access care [18,19].

This initial visit can also establish a trusting relationship between provider and client and is an opportunity to document baseline health measurements (weight, height, BMI, blood pressure) and to provide advice on weight gain during pregnancy. See Table 3 for specific pregnancy weight gain recommendations based on BMI.

The initial prenatal visit is also an opportunity to address the specific complications that can have a significant impact on the health of the pregnant person and fetus. These complications include:

- Diabetes
- Gestational hypertension
- Preeclampsia
- Medically indicated preterm birth
- Obstructive sleep apnea
- Fetal complications

Gestational diabetes. Type 2 and gestational diabetes mellitus are common in those affected by obesity and can have an impact on pregnancy outcomes. This

Table 3
Pregnancy weight gain recommendations

Weight gain recommendations for singleton pregnancy based on prepregnancy BMI	
BMI<18.5 kg/m^2	13–18 kg (28–40 pounds)
BMI 18.5–24.9 kg/m^2	11–16 kg (25–35 pounds)
BMI 25.0–29.9 kg/m^2	7–11 kg (15–25 pounds)
BMI 35 kg/m^2 and greater	5–9 kg (11–20 pounds)

risk increases as BMI increases and is related to an increase in insulin resistance that is inherent in clients with obesity [20]. It is therefore important to offer early glucose tolerance testing (typically with a 1-hour glucose tolerance test) and repeat testing for diabetes throughout the pregnancy. Table 1 provides specific information about glucose testing in pregnancy.

Gestational hypertension and preeclampsia. An increased BMI is also a risk factor for developing gestational hypertension and preeclampsia. One systematic review of 13 cohort studies reported that the risk of preeclampsia doubled with each increase of 5 to 7 kg/m^2 in BMI [21]. As with many complications of increased BMI, the mechanism that leads to hypertensive disorders in pregnancy are not well understood, but, like spontaneous abortion and diabetes, hypertension in pregnancy may be related to insulin resistance, hyperlipidemia, hormonal changes, and subclinical inflammation [22,23]. Clients affected by obesity should be offered baseline laboratory screening for preeclampsia in the form of urinalysis for protein and creatinine clearance along with liver function tests [22]. These laboratory tests should be repeated with any developing signs of preeclampsia.

Preterm birth. People with an increased BMI are also at higher risk of medically indicated preterm birth, largely because of complications such as hypertension, preeclampsia, and diabetes during pregnancy. These risks increase as BMI increases and can lead to interventions, medically necessary induction of labor, and preterm delivery. However, it is unclear whether patients affected by obesity are more likely to experience spontaneous preterm birth [24].

Sleep apnea. Obstructive sleep apnea is another complication of increased BMI that affects some individuals and can have an impact on pregnancy. Although most screening tools for sleep apnea are not validated for pregnant people and have not been shown to help guide providers, 1 recent tool is promising [25]. If a client is experiencing clear symptoms or complications associated with sleep apnea, a referral to a sleep specialist and further testing is warranted [25]. With few screening tools available, it is clear that more research is needed to provide better awareness and screening opportunities for obstructive sleep apnea in pregnancy.

Birth defects. In addition to these risk factors for pregnant individuals, there are associated fetal risks, including an increase in birth defects [26]. Specifically, those pregnancies carry a higher risk of cardiac, genitourinary, craniofacial, and neural tube anomalies [26]. Those risks increase as BMI increases [27], so patients of all sizes should have a discussion of personal risk factors, and, together with their prenatal providers, discuss what antenatal testing is appropriate and desired. This testing can include first trimester screening, targeted (level 2) ultrasonography, as well as more invasive testing such as chorionic villi sampling and amniocentesis. Some risk factors are well documented; however, there continues to be some debate as to whether patients affected with obesity should take a high-dose regimen of folic acid both preconceptually and antenatally. Although there is an increased risk for neural tube defects (NTDs) in obese populations, that risk is likely associated with undiagnosed diabetes. Regardless of the cause of NTD, the CDC currently recommends 400 µg of folic acid for patients with a BMI more than 25 kg/m^2 [26].

Reducing bias in pregnancy care

People with obesity have historically experienced stigma and bias from social interactions, including within the health care system. This situation is also the case when the person is pregnant and is experiencing challenges with stigma and bias during prenatal care [28]. It is hypothesized that the negative bias toward pregnant people with obesity may contribute to the poor outcomes that are increased in this patient population [28]. The stigma surrounding the diagnosis of obesity can be seen in past recommendations, where pregnancy care was more focused on intervention if the patient had a BMI more than 30 kg/m^2. The previous recommendations that are no longer considered to be evidence-based practice for this patient population include avoiding pregnancy if the person is more than 35 years old, urinalysis at each prenatal visit, and monthly growth ultrasonography scans throughout pregnancy. The current recommendations for prenatal care for people with BMI greater than 40 kg/m^2 focus on collaboration between low-risk and high-risk providers, and this trend toward collaborative practices has improved patient outcomes [7,29,30].

Because of this history of bias, it is important to consider the language that is used by providers who care for this population. The words used during antenatal care can influence the relationship between the patient and provider when negative bias is perceived by the client. For example, use of terms such as body fat and superobese are common in clinical parlance but can be seen as judgmental and insensitive. There are also moments when the biases are not as blatant (implicit bias). Implicit bias occurs when the thoughts and feelings about a certain population (eg, race, gender, body size) affect the person's actions subconsciously [31]. Implicit bias is present in everyone and can be addressed in the health care setting by training providers and staff to be aware of these existing beliefs. Implicit bias can affect the care provided to patients and damage the trust in the provider-patient relationship [32]. Health care providers should also be aware that there can even be poor patient outcomes caused by implicit bias in health care [32]. An important component of implicit bias is that it can be confronted and changed [31]. From hospital systems to individual clinics, health care systems are investing in implicit bias training to improve awareness about these harmful unconscious associations.

Table 4
Breaking down people-first language

Condition-first language	People-first language
Focus is on the medical condition	Focus is on the person instead of condition
Can promote bias	Promotes recognition of bias
Generalizes care	Individualizes care
Can lead to patient dissatisfaction	Promotes patient satisfaction
Can be divisive	Inclusive, not divisive
Past model taught in nursing and medical schools	Now used in medical education and is recognized in current medical literature
"This is an obese pregnant patient"	"This is a pregnant person with obesity"
"The disabled"	"People with disabilities"
"Autistic"	"Has autism"
"Obese woman"	"Woman with obesity"
"Diabetic man"	"Man with diabetes"

Negative attitudes toward people with obesity are common implicit biases. One way to combat the effects of this bias in health care is to choose people-first language. People-first language seeks to emphasize the "individuality, equality and dignity of people" [33] and "conveys respect by emphasizing the fact that people with disabilities are first and foremost just that–people" [33]. According to the Obesity Action Coalition (a group focused on supporting and empowering people affected by obesity through education and advocacy), using terms such as fat, obese, and extremely obese can feel stigmatizing to the individual, and affect their trust in the provider. In contrast, using less biased, inclusive, people-first language can allow positive, productive discussions about weight and health [34]. Table 4 gives examples of the differences in people-first versus condition-first language.

SUMMARY AND IMPLICATIONS FOR PRACTICE

The potential risks of pregnancy complicated by obesity are well documented, but management of these pregnancies has changed significantly in recent years [7]. Historically, a diagnosis of obesity meant a pregnant person risked out of low-risk models, such as nurse-midwifery care and family practice obstetrics. This exclusion is not always the case presently, and the choice of care model is often patient driven. In addition, the increase in the number of advanced practice registered nurses in America has led to an increase in certified nurse-midwives, women's health nurse practitioners, and FNPs who encounter pregnant patients with obesity within their practices.

Patients with the diagnosis of pregnancy and obesity are increasing in numbers in the United States and may see their primary care providers before prenatal care can be initiated. They may also choose to see their primary care providers throughout much of their pregnancies. FNPs should know the latest recommendations for pregnant patients with obesity in order to provide early prenatal care and then transfer each patient to a pregnancy provider when appropriate. Establishing a positive relationship with a client can help build trust and enhance the pregnant person's ability to make healthy choices, so it is important that FNPs are able to acknowledge biases held toward this patient population by both society and health care professionals.

CLINICS CARE POINTS

- Provider bias about obesity can negatively impact prenatal care.
- The first prenatal care visit is an opportunity to assess risks in pregnancy associated with obesity, but not all pregnant people with obesity will have a "high risk" pregnancy.
- A evidence-based and systematic checklist can direct care and ensure consistency across patient populations.

Disclosure

The authors have nothing to disclose.

References

[1] American College of Obstetricians and Gynecologists. ACOG committee opinion. Washington, DC: American College of Obstetricians and Gynecologists; 1978.

[2] CDC. Prevalence and trends in Prepregnancy Normal weight — 48 States, New York City, and District of Columbia, 2011–2015. 2018. Available at: https://www.cdc.gov/mmwr/volumes/66/wr/mm665152a3.htm. Accessed October 10, 2020.

[3] Chu SY, Callaghan WM, Kim SY, et al. Maternal obesity and risk of gestational diabetes mellitus. Diabetes care 2007;30(8):2070–6.

[4] Hales CM, Fryar CD, Carroll MD, et al. Trends in obesity and severe obesity prevalence in US youth and adults by sex and age, 2007-2008 to 2015-2016. Jama 2018;319(16):1723–5.

[5] PRAMS (2017). Available at: https://www.cdc.gov/prams/prams-data/mch-indicators/states/pdf/Selected-2016-2017-MCH-Indicators-Aggregate-by-Site_508.pdf. Accessed October 10, 2020.

[6] CDC, 2010.

[7] Reither M, Germano E, DeGrazia M. Midwifery Management of Pregnant Women Who Are Obese. J Midwifery Womens Health 2018;63(3):273–82.

[8] Lima & Mahmood. 2015.

[9] CDC. Adult obesity causes and Consequences 2020. Available at: https://www.cdc.gov/obesity/adult/causes.html.

[10] Centers for Disease Control and Prevention. Folic acid. 2019. Available at: https://www.cdc.gov/folicacid/recommendations.html. Accessed October 10, 2020.

[11] CDC. Weight gain during pregnancy. 2019. Available at: https://www.cdc.gov/reproductivehealth/maternalinfanthealth/pregnancy-weight-gain.htm#recommendations. Accessed October 10, 2020.

[12] Santos S, Voerman E, Amiano P. Impact of maternal body mass index and gestational weight gain on pregnancy complications. BJOG 2019;126(984):984–95.

[13] Cavalcante MB, Sarno M, Peixoto AB, et al. Obesity and recurrent miscarriage: A systematic review and meta-analysis. J Obstet Gynaecol Res 2018;45(1):30–8.

[14] Bellver J, Melo MA, Bosch E, et al. Obesity and poor reproductive outcome: The potential role of the endometrium. Fertil Steril 2007;88(2):446–51.

[15] Schummers L, Hutcheon JA, Bodnar LM, et al. Risk of adverse pregnancy outcomes by prepregnancy body mass index. Obstet Gynecol 2015;125(1):133–43.

[16] Jain AP, Gavard JA, Rice JJ, et al. The impact of interpregnancy weight change on birthweight in obese women. Obstet Gynecol Surv 2013;68(6):409–11.

[17] Sandall J, Soltani H, Gates S, et al. Midwife-led continuity models versus other models of care for childbearing women. Cochrane Database Syst Rev 2015; https://doi.org/10.1002/14651858.cd004667.pub4.

[18] ACOG Committee Opinion No 743 (2018). Low-dose Aspirin Use during pregnancy. Available at: https://www.acog.org/en/Clinical/Clinical%20Guidance/Committee%20Opinion/Articles/2018/07/Low-Dose%20Aspirin%20Use%20During%20Pregnancy. Accessed October 10, 2020.

[19] ACOG Committee Opinion No. 757. Screening for Perinatal Depression. Obstet Gynecol 2018;132(5); https://doi.org/10.1097/aog.0000000000002927.

[20] Kongubol A, Phupong V. Prepregnancy obesity and the risk of gestational diabetes mellitus. BMC Pregnancy Childbirth 2011;11(1); https://doi.org/10.1186/1471-2393-11-59.

[21] O'Brien TE, Ray JG, Chan W. Maternal body mass index and the risk of preeclampsia: a systematic overview. Epidemiology 2003;14(3):368–74.

[22] Wolf M, Kettyle E, Sandler L, et al. Obesity and Preeclampsia. Obstet Gynecol 2001;98(5, Part 1):757–62.

[23] Zheng Y, Shen Y, Jiang S, et al. Maternal glycemic parameters and adverse pregnancy outcomes among high-risk pregnant women. BMJ Open Diabetes Res Care 2019;7(1): e000774.

[24] Mcdonald S, Han Z, Mulla S, et al. Overweight and obesity in mothers and risk of preterm birth and low birth weight infants. Obstet Anesth Dig 2011;31(3):158–9.

[25] Izci-Balserak B, Zhu B, Gurubhagavatula I, et al. A screening Algorithm for obstructive sleep apnea in pregnancy. 2019. Available at: https://www.ncbi.nlm.nih.gov/pubmed/31162952. Accessed September 01, 2020.

[26] Correa A, Marcinkevage J. Prepregnancy obesity and the risk of birth defects: an update. Nutr Rev 2013;71(suppl_1):S68–77.

[27] Watkins ML, Rasmussen SA, Honein MA, et al. Maternal obesity and risk for birth defects. Pediatrics 2003;111(Supplement 1):1152–8.

[28] DeJoy S, Bittner K. Obesity stigma as a determinant of poor birth outcomes in women with high BMI: a conceptual framework. Matern Child Health J 2015;19(4):693–9.

[29] Carlson NS, Breman R, Neal JL, et al. Preventing cesarean birth in women with obesity: influence of unit-level midwifery presence on use of cesarean among women in the Consortium on Safe Labor data set. J Midwifery Womens Health 2020;65(1):22–32.

[30] Centers for Disease Control (CDC). Defining Adult overweight and obesity. 2020. Available at: https://www.cdc.gov/obesity/adult/defining.html. Accessed October 10, 2020.

[31] The Kirwan Institute for the Study of Race and Ethnicity. Understanding implicit bias. Ohio State University. 2015. Available at: http://kirwaninstitute.osu.edu/research/understanding-implicit-bias/#:~:text=Also%20known%20as%20implicit%20social,decisions%20in%20an%20unconscious%20manner. Accessed October 10, 2020.

[32] Tomiyama AJ, Carr D, Granberg EM, et al. How and why weight stigma drives the obesity 'epidemic' and harms health. BMC Med 2018;16(1):123.

[33] EARN Employee Assistance Resource Network. 2020. Available at: https://askearn.org/. Accessed August 27, 2020.

[34] Puhl RM, Phelan SM, Nadglowski J, et al. Overcoming weight bias in the management of patients with diabetes and obesity. Clin Diabetes 2016;34(1):44–50.

CONSIDERATIONS FOR PROVIDING PRENATAL CARE FOR PREGNANT PATIENTS WITH OBESITY

BMI 25 to 29.9 kg/m^2, overweight
- Preconceptual counseling on weight loss with goal of BMI less than 25 kg/m^2
- Recommend daily prenatal vitamin with 400 μg of folic acid, ideally started 3 months before conception
- Counsel total weight gain should be 7 to 11 (15–25 pounds)
- In-office education about diet and exercise in pregnancy
- Discuss optional screening tests available for birth defects (nuchal translucency or noninvasive prenatal testing)
- Level 1 ultrasonography at or around 20 weeks
- Glucose screening in first trimester based on individual risk
- Glucose screening at 28 weeks
- Growth sonograms as indicated for individual needs

BMI 30 to 34.9 kg/m^2, class I obesity
- Preconception counseling on weight loss with goal of BMI less than 25 kg/m^2 or at least 10% weight loss before conception
- Recommend daily prenatal vitamin with 400 μg of folic acid, ideally started 3 months before conception
- Baby aspirin (ASA) (81 mg) daily starting at 12 weeks
- Counsel total weight gain 5 to 9 kg (11–20 pounds)
- Offer nutrition consult
- Discuss optional screening tests available for birth defects
- Level 2 ultrasonography at or around 20 weeks
- Glucose screening in first and third trimester and as needed
- Growth sonogram in the third trimester and as needed

BMI 35 to 39.9 kg/m^2, class II obesity
- Preconception counseling on weight loss with goal of BMI less than 25 kg/m^2 or at least 10% weight loss before conception
- Recommend daily prenatal vitamin with 400 μg of folic acid ideally started 3 months before conception
- Baby ASA daily starting at 12 weeks
- Consider baseline laboratory tests for preeclampsia in second trimester and as needed
- Counsel total weight gain of 5 to 9 kg (11–20 pounds)
- Recommend nutrition consult
- Consider maternal-fetal medicine (MFM) consult
- Discuss optional screening tests for birth defects
- Screening or targeted sonogram at or around 20 weeks, consider fetal echocardiogram
- Glucose screening in first and third trimester and as needed

- Growth sonogram in the third trimester, consider serial growth as needed
- Consider antenatal fetal surveillance (nonstress test [NST]/biophysical profile [BPP] at regular intervals) in the third trimester because of increased risk of poor placental perfusion and stillbirth
- Counsel patient on risk of increased stillbirth risk with higher BMI and provide informed consent for patient if delivery at term is recommended

BMI greater than or equal to 40 kg/m^2, class III obesity

- Preconception counseling on weight loss with goal of less than 25 kg/m^2 or at least 10% weight loss before conception
- Recommend daily prenatal vitamin with 400 µg of folic acid, ideally started 3 months before conception
- Baby ASA daily starting at 12 weeks
- Consider baseline laboratory tests for preeclampsia in second trimester and as needed
- Counsel total weight gain of 5 to 9 kg (11–20 pounds)
- Recommend nutrition consult
- Recommend MFM consult
- Discuss optional screening for birth defects, recommend targeted sonogram with fetal echocardiogram
- Level 2 ultrasonography at or around 20 weeks
- Glucose screening in first and third trimester and as needed
- Serial growth ultrasonography scans beginning at 28 weeks and continuing every 3 to 4 weeks until delivery
- Antenatal surveillance starting between 32 and 36 weeks, including NST and BPP at least weekly
- Delivery at term

Deciphering Pap Guidelines and Determining Management in Primary Care

Mary Lauren Pfieffer, DNP, FNP-BC*,
Lacey Cross, MSN, FNP-BC¹

Vanderbilt University School of Nursing, 461 21st Avenue South, Nashville, TN 37240, USA

Keywords
- Cervical cancer • Cervical cancer screening
- Cervical cancer screening guidelines • Cervical cancer treatment
- Human papillomavirus (HPV)

Key points
- Cervical cancer is a leading cause of cancer worldwide. When screened appropriately, it can be preventable. It is also very treatable when caught in early stages.
- Human papillomavirus (HPV) has been shown to cause the majority of cervical cancers. Therefore, in 2012, HPV cotesting was added to diagnostic testing for cervical cancer.
- The initial cervical cancer screening is age 21 and then performed at intervals based on age.
- Treatment of cervical cancer is based on cervical/endocervical cytology and HPV results but can include coloscopy, cone biopsy, excisional treatment, cryotherapy, hysterectomy, and thermal ablation.
- Health promotion to prevent cervical cancer includes encouraging HPV vaccine in patients ages 12 to 26, including education on completing vaccine series.

INTRODUCTION
Cervical cancer is one of the leading causes of cancer in women worldwide [1]. Over the past 30 years, the United States as seen a downward trend in the incidence and mortality rate of cervical cancer. This downward trend is

¹Present address: 522 Inwood Drive. Nashville. TN 3721122.

*Corresponding author. 9235 Brushboro Drive, Brentwood, TN 37027. E-mail address: mary.pfieffer@vanderbilt.edu

https://doi.org/10.1016/j.yfpn.2021.01.009
2589-420X/21/© 2021 Elsevier Inc. All rights reserved.

attributable in part to the increasing rates of cervical cancer screening and detection in the United States during this time period. The National Cancer Institute (NCI) reports that in 1990 there was an observed rate of 10.7 new cases of cervical cancer per 100,000 individuals, with a mortality rate of 3.5% [2]. Data from 2017 indicate an observed new case rate of 6.6 per 100,000 individuals, with a mortality rate of 2.2% [2]. Current NCI estimates suggest 13,800 new cases were detected in the United States in 2020 [2].

Technology for detecting these cancers is constantly evolving, resulting in the development of multiple screening strategies performed at various intervals [3]. Dr George Papanicolaou introduced cervical cytology reviewing cellular morphology in 1943 with the Papanicolaou (Pap) smear [4]. An improvement in cervical cancer screenings occurred in 1996 with the creation of thin-layer technology cervical screenings called ThinPrep Pap Test (Cytyc Corp., Box-borough, Massachusetts) [4]. ThinPrep improved diagnosis of cervical cancers drastically [4]. Recommendations for appropriate screening intervals and management of screening results also frequently are changing, presenting a challenge to providers who recommend and perform screening and also creating confusion among patients regarding the timing and necessity of screenings.

Cervical cancer largely is preventable and when detected early also can be very treatable. Human papillomavirus (HPV) has been identified as a leading cause of cervical cancer in women with persistent infection. It is estimated that prior to the vaccine era, 80% of individuals acquired HPV during their lifetime, often by age 45 [5]. The advent of the HPV vaccine has reduced the rate of infection with this sexually transmitted virus, subsequently reducing rates of cervical cancer by up to approximately 2% annually [6]. Despite the progress made in prevention and early identification of cervical cancer, this remains the fourth most common cancer diagnosis in women worldwide [7]. Therefore, adequate screening and management of patients remain essential to the overall health promotion of the female population.

HISTORY

Cancer of the cervix often is asymptomatic in the early stages of disease, making it difficult to detect without routine screening until the disease has become advanced, when prognosis generally is poor [7]. In patients who do present with early symptoms, these most commonly include irregular vaginal bleeding or bleeding that is heavier than normal, especially after intercourse [6]. Patients also may complain of vaginal discharge, which may be malodorous [6,7]. See Table 1 for a list of differential diagnoses. Symptoms of advanced disease

Table 1			
Differential diagnoses for vaginal bleeding, discharge, and odor [8,9]			
Cervical cancer	Cervical inflammation	Endometriosis	Postcoital bleeding
Cervical ectropion	Cervical polyps	Mesonephric cysts	Sexually transmitted infections
Cervical fibroids	Cervicitis	Nabothian cysts	

may include pain in the pelvis or lower back, sometimes radiating to the posterior lower extremities [6]. Providers also should evaluate for the presence of any bowel or bladder symptoms, such as hematuria, the passage of any urine or stool through the vagina, and hematochezia, because these also can indicate severe disease [6]. Additionally, the presence of constitutional symptoms, such as unintentional weight changes, fatigue, and malaise, also should be reviewed.

Providers also should assess prior medical history as well as risk factors for cervical cancer (Table 2). Additionally, providers should evaluate surgical history, especially for hysterectomy, because women who have had total hysterectomy with cervix removal who do not have a history of cervical cancer or high-grade precancerous lesions do not require screening [10]. Those who have had subtotal hysterectomy with any remaining cervical tissue should continue to be screened. Number of sexual partners increases cervical cancer risk. Cervical cancer risk doubles with 2 partners and risk triples with 6 partners or more [6].

PATHOPHYSIOLOGY

HPV is a known predominant cause of cervical cancer worldwide, and HPV DNA is present in more than 99% of cervical cancers across the globe [6]. HPV strains are classified as high risk or low risk based on their oncogenic properties [11]. At least 14 strains have been identified as high risk, and 2 strands (16 and 18) account for a significant percentage of cervical cancer diagnoses [11]. In cervical cancer, HPV invades cells of the cervix and over time triggers uncontrolled cell growth resulting in malignancy [11].

Both malignant and premalignant lesions most often originate at the squamo-columnar junction of the cervical canal, also known as the transformation zone [11]. Cytologic evaluation involves inspection of cells collected from this region for any cellular changes that may suggest abnormality. Some malignant lesions are noticeable on visual examination of the cervix during a pelvic examination, whereas others may be identified only through cytology testing. Suspicious lesions should be evaluated with cytology and/or biopsy to identify the presence of abnormal cells.

ASSESSMENT

Assessment starts with examination of the external genitalia then moves to lymph nodes in the inguinal area. Then the speculum is inserted to visualize

Table 2			
Risk factors [6,7]			
Sexual Debut before age 18	More than 1 sexual partner	High-risk sexual partners	Immunosuppression
History of HIV	History of other STIs	History of HPV	Previous abnormal Pap smears
Smoking history	Parity	DES exposure	Prolonged oral contraceptive use

the cervix and vaginal vault. The collection of the Pap smear occurs next as specimens for both cervical cytology and HPV testing are collected from the cervix. Cervical cytology and HPV testing not always are tested together, because it depends on the ability of diagnostic testing and age of patient. After collecting cervical cytology, remove the speculum and do a bimanual examination to assess for any palpable abnormalities [7].

There are several expert societies within the United States that have established guidelines for cervical cancer screening in the general population, including which tests should be performed at which intervals. These guidelines for routine screening are applicable to individuals who are asymptomatic and not currently under surveillance for previously abnormal results. The 3 main guidelines are those from the American Cancer Society (ACS)/American Society for Colposcopy and Cervical Pathology (ASCCP)/American Society for Clinical Pathology (ASCP), the US Preventive Services Task Force (USPSTF), and American College of Obstetricians and Gynecologists (ACOG). The ACS published its own independent set of guidelines, in July 2020, which also are included in this review.

SCREENING GUIDELINES
American Cancer Society/American Society for Colposcopy and Cervical Pathology/American Society for Clinical Pathology
In 2012, the ACS, ASCCP, and ASCP published joint guidelines for cervical cancer screening (Table 3). These guidelines indicate that screening in patients under age 21 is not indicated [12]. For patients ages 21 to 29, screening should include cytology testing only every 3 years [12]. Beginning at age 30 and through age 65, cotesting every 5 years is the preferred method but cytology alone every 3 years is acceptable [12]. When the 2012 ACS/ASCCP/ASCP joint guideline initially was published, it included recommendation against the use of high-risk HPV (hrHPV) testing in isolation. These 3 organizations, however, subsequently released a new interim guideline for the use of this testing method in 2015, suggesting that hrHPV alone is an acceptable alternative when performed in women over age 25 at least every 5 years but not more frequently than every 3 years [13]. Screening may be discontinued after age 65 if patients have had adequate negative prior screening [12].

The US Preventive Services Task Force
The USPSTF published an updated statement most recently in 2018 (see Table 3). Generally, the USPSTF recommends that patients between ages 21 and 29 should be screened every 3 years with cervical cytology testing alone [10]. For patients between 30 years and 65 years, the USPSTF recommends 3 possible options for screening: every 3 years with cytology alone, every 5 years with cotesting, or every 5 years with hrHPV testing alone [10]. Screening is not recommended in patients ages 65 and older who have had prior adequate screening nor is it recommended in patients younger than 21 years [10]. These recommendations apply only to individuals who have a cervix, and do not

Table 3
Screening guidelines by organization [3,10,12–14]

	Ages under 21 years	Ages 21 years to 29 years	Ages 30 year to 65 years	Ages older than 65 years
ACS/ ASCCP/ ASCP (2012)	Screening not recommended	Cytology every 3 y May begin HPV testing every 5 y at age 25 y	Cytology every 3 y Cotesting every 5 y Primary HPV testing every 5 y	Discontinue screening if prior adequate screening has been confirmed.
ACS (2020)	Screening not recommended	Initiate screening at age 25 y with primary HPV testing every 5 y. May utilize cytology every 3 y OR cotesting every 5 y	Primary HPV testing every 5 y (preferred) Cytology every 3 y Cotesting every 5 y	Discontinue screening if prior adequate screening has been confirmed.
USPSTF (2018)	Screening not recommended	Cytology every 3 y	Cytology every 3 y Cotesting every 5 y Primary HPV testing every 5 y	Discontinue screening if prior adequate screening has been confirmed.
ACOG (2016)	Screening not recommended	Cytology every 5 y	Cytology every 3 y Cotesting every 5 y	Discontinue screening if prior adequate screening has been confirmed.

apply to patients who have been diagnosed with a high-grade precancerous lesion or cervical cancer, immunocompromised patients, or those who were exposed to diethylstilbestrol in utero [10].

American College of Obstetricians and Gynecologists

The ACOG published a set of guidelines in 2016 that are similar to those set forth by the USPSTF (see Table 3). ACOG recommends against screening before 21 years of age except for those who are immunocompromised or have HIV [3]. Like the other groups discussed previously, ACOG recommends screening every 3 years with cytology alone in patients ages 21 to 29 and specifically recommend against cotesting in this age group [3]. In women ages 30 to 65, ACOG recommends cotesting with cytology and hrHPV testing every 5 years as the preferred method but states cytology alone every 3 years is acceptable [3]. In their 2016 bulletin, ACOG does not make their own recommendation with regard to hrHPV testing alone but defers to the joint interim guidelines set forth on this topic in 2015 by the ACS, ASCCP, and ASCP. ACOG recommends that screening be discontinued after age 65 as long as prior adequate screening has been confirmed and there is no history of cervical intraepithelial neoplasia grade 2 (CIN 2) or higher lesion [3]. Adequate screening is defined as 3 negative cytology results or 2 negative cotesting results within the past 10 years [3].

American Cancer Society 2020 updates

In July 2020, the ACS published updated guidelines for screening, which contain new recommendations compared with the 2012 joint guidelines published collaboratively with ASCCP and ASCP (see Table 3). ACS now recommends initiation of screening at age 25, not age 21 [14]. There is relatively high rate of HPV infection in women age 21 to 24 but frequent natural regression of transient infection and associated low-grade lesions [14]. Screening and treating patients in this age group have resulted in minimal reduction of invasive disease and perhaps overtreatment and potential harm to patients who have undergone invasive procedures for management [14].

The ACS's preferred method and interval for screening is primary HPV testing every 5 years, beginning at age 25 and continuing through age 65, at which time screening may be discontinued if adequate prior screening has been confirmed [14]. The ACS continues to accept cotesting every 5 years or cytology alone every 3 years as adequate screening methods, although they predict a transition from cytology-based screening toward primary HPV screening in the coming years, especially as primary HPV screening becomes more widely available [14].

These new guidelines from the ACS differ from the guidelines published by other organizations like USPSTF and ACOG, which largely are consistent with each other in their screening recommendations. The USPSTF most recently published guidelines in 2018 and ACOG did so in 2016. Clinicians should remain aware of the evolving recommendations among organizations, especially with regard to the predicted transition to primary HPV screening.

DIAGNOSIS

A definitive diagnosis of cervical cancer is made through histologic evaluation of cervical tissue [6]. When abnormal cellular changes are identified with cervical cytology or when hrHPV DNA is detected in cervical cell specimens, patients often undergo additional testing, which may include colposcopy with biopsy [15]. The determination regarding which additional testing is required is dependent on the which cytologic changes or HPV strains are detected. Some abnormal results warrant immediate biopsy whereas others are managed with repeat screening at more frequent intervals. There are 3 primary strategies for routine cervical cancer screening in the United States. These include stand-alone cervical cytology, primary HPV testing, and cotesting with cytology and HPV testing together [15].

DIAGNOSTIC TESTING

Cervical cancer diagnostic testing has changed drastically over the years to improve diagnosis and effect swifter treatment if necessary. The biggest changes to screenings have occurred in the past 20 years. Historically, cervical cancer was diagnosed through Pap smear testing. This cervical cell smear was fixed to a slide and then sent for traditional Pap staining [4]. This testing yielded high false-negative rates [4]. Thin-layer technology cervical screenings through ThinPrep Pap Test and other brands improved screenings. ThinPrep sampling included a broom sampling device or a spatula/cytobrush combination [4]. The cervical sample was rinsed into a fixed solution vial and sent to laboratory [4]. Once in the laboratory, the vial is processed, and cells are collected on a filter, which then go onto slides [4]. These slides then are sent for traditional Pap staining [4]. Thin-layer technology screenings still are performed today and continue to be superior to traditional Pap smears. Cytologic testing can identify various cellular abnormalities, and results currently are reported using the Bethesda classification system that was developed in 1988 and most recently revised in 2014 (Table 4) [16].

HPV has been shown to cause a majority of cervical cancers [18]. Therefore in 2012, HPV cotesting was added to diagnostic testing for cervical cancer. HPV cotesting uses the same cervical cell sample as the thin-layer technology. HPV is diagnosed by the presence of nucleic acid in the cervical cells [19]. Most of the tests are designed to detect the 14 most common hrHPV strains [3]. HPV testing has a higher sensitivity to detecting precancers than the thin-layer technology [19]. It does, however, have less specificity alone than cytology in identifying patients at risk for invasive cervical cancer [12]. Until recently, stand-alone HPV testing as primary screening for cervical cancer was not accepted as an effective method for cervical cancer screening and HPV previously was performed only as part of cotesting with cytology. There is now increasing evidence, however, to suggest that primary HPV testing is an acceptable and effective screening alternative [13]. Guidance first was published to direct clinicians on its use in 2015 and has been updated to reflect changes in result management in 2020 [15].

Table 4
Bethesda terminology for cervical cytology [16,17]

Acronym	Cytology result
ASC-H	Atypical squamous cells, cannot exclude HSIL
ASCUS	Atypical squamous cells of undetermined significance
HSIL	High-grade squamous intraepithelial lesion
LSIL	Low-grade squamous intraepithelial lesion
NILM	Negative for intraepithelial lesion or malignancy

MANAGEMENT

Screening intervals are based on patient age and previous cytology history. The initial cervical cancer screening is age 21. This recommendation is related to exceptionally low cervical cancer rates in this age group [20]. Once the initial screening is completed, then patients initiate age-based recommendations.

Ages 21 to 24 years

Guidelines indicate performing cervical cytology alone every 3 years in this age group [17,21]. HPV cotesting is not recommended because incidental HPV infection occurs frequently in this age group [17]. Management is based on results.

Ages 25 years to 29 years

Frequency guidelines remain the same for this age group as they do for ages 21 to 24, the changes are seen in the management. Patients ages 25 to 29 should have cervical cytology alone every 3 years [17,21]. HPV cotesting is not recommended. Management is based on results.

Ages 30 years to 65 years

Guidelines indicate that women ages 30 to 65 need to have cervical cytology and hrHPV testing (cotesting) performed every 5 years [10,21–23]. Some guidelines suggest an alternative is cervical cytology alone every 3 years [21]. Management is based on results.

Ages 65 years and older

Women over the age of 65 who have had negative screenings can cease Pap smears. These patients need to have had 3 consecutive negative cytology results or 2 consecutive negative cotesting results [17,20,21]. Cervical cancer incidence is low in patients who have a history of regular negative screenings [20,21].

History of hysterectomy

Patients who are post-hysterectomy potentially can cease cervical cancer screenings, but it depends on the reasoning behind hysterectomy. If patients did not have cervical dysplasia, they do not need a screening after complete hysterectomy [17,25]. If patients had hysterectomy related to cervical dysplasia or cervical cancer, the patient needs to continue vaginal cytology for 20 years post-hysterectomy [17,25].

TREATMENT

Treatment is based on cervical/endocervical cytology and HPV results (Tables 5–7). When reviewing the results, health care providers are assessing likelihood of cells progressing into invasive cervical cancer [17]. Historically, conization and hysterectomy were mainstays of treatment, but colposcopy radically changed treatment algorithms and improved patient outcomes [21,26]. The various treatments options are discussed later.

Table 5
Screening guidelines for ages 21 years to 24 years [21–24]

Cytology result	Management
Normal	Repeat Pap smear in 3 y
Unsatisfactory	Repeat cytology in 2–4 mo
ASCUS	Repeat Pap smear in 12 mo OR perform a reflex HPV test on current Pap smear
ASC-H	Colposcopy
LSIL	Repeat Pap smear in 12 mo
HSIL	Colposcopy

*Reminder that HPV testing is not necessary for the 21-year to 24-year age group.

Colposcopy

Colposcopy is performed with a colposcope, which has an intricate lens system that allows for close evaluation of cervix [26]. Colposcopes looks specifically at the transformation zone of the cervix [26]. Colposcopy can identify many types of cellular changes that lead to cervical cancer: intraepithelial neoplasia, squamous intraepithelial lesions (atypical squamous cells of undetermined significance [ASCUS]; atypical squamous cells, cannot exclude high-grade SIL [ASC-H]; low-grade squamous intraepithelial lesion [LSIL]; and high-grade squamous intraepithelial lesion [HSIL]) and invasive cervical cancer [26]. During the colposcopy, a 3% to 5% acetic-acid solution is applied to area and visual changes are assessed [17]. Biopsies can be taken at the same time as a colposcopy. Excisional procedures also can be performed during encounter [26]. Providers who can perform colposcopies are called colposcopists and they need specific training and clinical preparation (Khan and colleagues, 2017). The risks of colposcopies are low but include bleeding and infection [26]. Colposcopies can be performed during pregnancy and the risks are low. If there is a colposcopy performed during pregnancy, there is follow-up postpartum.

Table 6
Screening guidelines for ages 25 years to 29 years [21–24]

Cytology result	Management
Normal	Repeat Pap smear in 3 y
Unsatisfactory	Repeat cytology in 2–4 mo
ASCUS	Repeat Pap smear in 12 mo OR perform a reflex HPV test on current Pap smear
ASC-H	Colposcopy
LSIL	Colposcopy
HSIL	Colposcopy or excisional treatment

*Reminder that HPV testing is not necessary for the 25-year to 29-year age group.

Table 7
Screening guidelines for ages 30 years to 65 years [21–24]

Cytology result	Management
Normal	HPV negative—cotesting every 5 y or cytology every 3 y
	HPV positive—cotesting in 12 mo or HPV typing
Unsatisfactory	HPV negative—repeat cytology in 2–4 mo
	HPV positive—colposcopy
ASCUS	HPV negative—repeat cotesting in 3 y
	HPV positive—colposcopy
ASC-H	HPV negative—colposcopy
	HPV positive—colposcopy
LSIL	HPV negative—repeat Pap in 12 mo or colposcopy
	HPV positive—colposcopy
HSIL	HPV negative—excisional treatment or colposcopy
	HPV positive—excisional treatment or colposcopy

Cone biopsy

Cone biopsy also is known as cold knife cone (CKC) biopsy and conization. This treatment is used when there is moderate to high-grade cervical dysplasia [17]. A cone-shaped excision is made into the cervix to excise the cellular dysplasia, hence the name of the procedure [27]. Pathologists review excised cells during the procedure, which can ensure clear cervical cell margins [17]. Close surveillance is needed if margins are not clear. It is important for providers to consider if patients have good access to care to decide if this treatment method is appropriate for patient [27]. Risks for this procedure are subsequent preterm labors [17].

Cryotherapy

This modality of treatment was created in 1970s and greatly improved treatment options for abnormal cervical findings [21]. This treatment includes use of a cryoprobe that is applied to area of cervical dysplasia. This device is attached to either nitrogen dioxide or carbon dioxide [28]. The gas from the device causes tissue necrosis of surrounding tissue [28]. Cryotherapy is a great treatment option in lower resource settings related to limited equipment needed [29]. Side effects and risks for cryotherapy are minimal [29].

Excisional treatment

Excisional treatment is performed with the loop electrosurgical excision procedure. This procedure was developed in the 1990s [21]. The procedure uses electrical current to excise cervical dysplasia. It can be performed in office with local anesthesia, which is advantage to this treatment modality. [21] Similar to the CKC biopsy, a pathologist reviews samples to ensure clear margins

[17]. It is important that health care providers performing excisional procedures have specific training and clinical preparation. Risks for this procedure include subsequent miscarriages and preterm births [17,21].

Hysterectomy
Hysterectomy is an option for treatment of cervical cancer. Hysterectomies related to cancers confined to cervix have high cure rates [30]. There is current controversy on which method of hysterectomy is appropriate for treatment— open versus minimally invasive [30]. There are surgical related risks related to both types of hysterectomy procedures. Continued screening is recommended in this population related to potential for vaginal cancer [25].

Thermal ablation
This technology was developed in the 1960s as a means to eradicate intraepithelial neoplasia [31]. During this treatment, a probe heated to 100°C to 120°C is applied to the cervical lesion for 20 seconds to 45 seconds duration [31]. Side effects to thermal ablation are vaginal discharge, uterine cramping, and mild bleeding post-procedure [31]. Advantages of this procedure is that it is relatively easy to perform, although health care providers need specific training and clinical preparation.

REFERRALS
Cervical cancer screening often is performed in primary care. It is important for primary care providers to understand their scope limitations when managing cervical cytology and HPV status. Providers who perform colposcopies, CKC biopsy, cryotherapy, excisional treatment, and thermal ablation need specific training and clinical preparation. Often these procedures are performed by a women's health nurse practitioner, an obstetrician-gynecologist (OB-GYN), a certified nurse midwife (CNM), or a certified midwife (MW). Any provider performing these procedures would have special training. OB-GYNs are the providers who perform hysterectomies. Specifically, an oncology OB-GYN provides care if cervical cancer is present. Referring patients to the appropriate resources allows for swifter treatment and improved follow-up.

HEALTH PROMOTION
Avoiding HPV infection is the primary way to prevent cervical cancer screening [7]. HPV infection can be avoided through no sexual activity, accurate condom uses, or mutual monogamous relationships having with no history of other partners [7]. The only way to prevent HPV infection through primary prevention is with the recommended HPV vaccine series [7]. Receiving the vaccine series has shown a reduction in colposcopies and cervical therapies [32]. High-income countries have implemented this vaccine series and seen significant improvement in cervical cancer numbers, whereas low-income and lower-middle-income countries have not been as successful in implementing HPV vaccine [33]. The World Health Organization has taken an initiative to improve vaccine accessibility and cervical cancer eradication to

the low-income and lower-middle-income countries by the end of the century [33,34]. Recently, there has been an increase in HPV vaccine uptake which is encouraging for prevention [35].

Gardasil was the first vaccine approved for HPV prevention and it now has been replaced by Gardasil 9 related to better prevention of cervical intraepithelial neoplasia grade 3 (CIN 3) [32]. Cervarix is the other competing HPV vaccine. Both Gardasil9 and Cervarix are synthetically made and protect against HPV 16/HPV 18 [32]. HPV 16 is the most prevalent type of HPV that leads to cervical cancer [32]. Gardasil 9 also includes 7 additional HPV types to provide additional coverage. According to Harper and DeMars, "Three dose efficacy preventing CIN 2 or worse by any HPV type is about 62% for both Cervarix and Gardsail9; the three dose efficacy preventing CIN 3 or worse by any HPV type is 93% for Cervarix and 43% for Gardasil, with no data for Gardasil9" [32]. The World Health Organization and Centers for Disease Control and Prevention Advisory Committee on Immunization Practices recommend 2 doses of Cervarix or Gardasil9 before age 15, given 6 months apart. If patients start vaccine series after age 15 through age 26, they need a third HPV vaccine [32,36]. HPV vaccine can be given after age 26 through age 45, but insurance likely does not cover it because the reasoning is related to increased likelihood of exposure to HPV after age 26 [36].

Secondary prevention of cervical cancer is through the Pap smear and HPV cotesting [7]. Patients need to remain current with their cervical cancer screenings and remember which testing was performed on them if they change providers. HPV vaccines never should replace consistent Pap smear screenings. Screening guidelines can be confusing to decipher for patients and providers alike until familiarity occurs. Follow-up on abnormal Pap smear is important and time is an important factor. Consistent screenings have shown to detect precervical cancer and cervical cancer at earlier and treatable stages [37].

PATIENT EDUCATION

Globally cervical cancer is one of the leading causes of cancer morbidity and mortality [38]. Screening for cervical cancer is an important tool for prevention but patient knowledge is limited on current screening guidelines [39]. Many patients believe that yearly screenings still are recommended [39]. Patient education can improve this belief radically. Equipping patients with knowledge and evidence supporting current guidelines is paramount. This improves patients' understanding and allows health care providers to provide evidence-based screenings [39]. Health literacy needs to be considered with cervical cancer screening to ensure information is shared appropriately [39].

Patients do not need a cervical cancer screening until age 21. Performing these examinations earlier than necessary adds to increased patient anxiety and overall health care costs. Education supporting accurate examination timing is important for patient care. Preparing and educating patient in visits leading up to cervical cancer screening decrease anxiety and apprehension related to the examination.

Patient education also is important because vaccine nonadherence for the HPV series is a problem [40]. Issues with HPV vaccine compliance relate to many knowledge gaps of parents and patients [41]. Some families are apprehensive to the vaccine because HPV is related to sexual activity and they do not want to consent to sexual activity for their child [41]. Families also are concerned about adverse reactions of the vaccine, so education about side effects of vaccine can help dispel these doubts [40]. Cost is the last concern related to the HPV vaccine and, in the United States, the vaccine is covered through the Vaccines for Children program [40]. Patient education surrounding these specific concerns will improve HPV vaccine rates.

Patient education also needs to include the continuation of annual examinations after the cessation of Pap smears. Ensuring that women know they need to continue annual examinations is an important part of health promotion. Beginning this conversation several years before the cessation of Pap smears is important to allow patients to find other care providers if necessary.

The ASCCP has a phone application that can be downloaded to keep providers aware of guidelines and treatment recommendations. This application is updated frequently with guideline and management changes. It is called ASCCP Management Guidelines.

SUMMARY

Cervical cancer remains one of the leading causes of death for women worldwide, even with the downward trend in statistics related to the implementation of the HPV vaccine. It is important for providers to be up to date on current screening algorithms and management. This equips patients with knowledge to stay on top of cervical cancer screenings. Promptly referring when treatment is out of provider scope of practice is important for patient outcomes. Educating and implementing the HPV vaccine series for age-appropriate patients are important in clinical practice. Implementing appropriately timed cervical cancer screenings and HPV vaccines into clinical practice can improve the overall health promotion of the female patient population.

Disclosure

The authors have nothing to disclose.

References

[1] Small W Jr, Bacon MA, Bajaj A, et al. Cervical cancer: A global health crisis. Cancer 2017;123(13):2404–12.

[2] National Cancer Institute. Cancer stat facts: cervical cancer 2020. Available at: https://seer.cancer.gov/statfacts/html/cervix.html. Accessed June 22, 2020.

[3] Practice Bulletin No. 168: Cervical Cancer Screening and Prevention. Obstet Gynecol 2016;128(4):e111–30.

[4] Guidos BJ, Selvaggi SM. "Use of the thin prep pap test in clinical practice." Diagnostic cytopathology., vol.20. Igaku-Shoin Medical Publishers; 1999. p. 70–3; https://doi.org/10.1002/(SICI)1097-0339(199902)20:2<70::AID-DC5>3.0.CO;2-E, no. 2.

[5] Chesson HW, Dunne EF, Hariri S, et al. The estimated lifetime probability of acquiring human papillomavirus in the United States. Sex Transm Dis 2014;41(11):660–4.

[6] Johnson CA, James D, Marzan A, et al. Cervical cancer: an overview of pathophysiology and management. Semin Oncol Nurs 2019;35(2):166–74.

[7] Cohen PA, Jhingran A, Oaknin A, et al. Cervical cancer. Lancet 2019;393(10167): 169–82.

[8] Fowler JR, Jack BW. Cervical Cancer. [Updated 2020 Aug 11]. In: StatPearls [Internet]. Treasure Island (FL): StatPearls Publishing; 2020. p. 1–15, https://www. ncbi.nlm.nih.gov/books/NBK431093/#_NBK431093_pubdet.

[9] Frumovitz M. Invasive cervical cancer: epidemiology, risk factors, clinical manifestations, and diagnosis. In: Post T, editor. UpToDate. Waltham (MA): UpToDate; 2020. Available at: www.uptodate.com https://www.uptodate.com/contents/invasive-cervical-cancer-epidemiology-risk-factors-clinical-manifestations-and-diagnosis#H11. Accessed June 15, 2020.

[10] US Preventive Services Task Force. Screening for cervical cancer: us preventive services task force recommendation statement. JAMA 2018;320(7):674–86.

[11] Ibeanu OA. Molecular pathogenesis of cervical cancer. Cancer Biol Ther 2011;11(3): 295–306.

[12] Saslow D, Solomon D, Lawson HW, et al. American Cancer Society, American Society for Colposcopy and Cervical Pathology, and American Society for Clinical Pathology screening guidelines for the prevention and early detection of cervical cancer. CA Cancer J Clin 2012;62(3):147–72.

[13] Huh WK, Ault KA, Chelmow D, et al. Use of primary high-risk human papillomavirus testing for cervical cancer screening: interim clinical guidance. Obstet Gynecol 2015;125(2): 330–7.

[14] Fontham ETH, Wolf AMD, Church TR, et al. Cervical cancer screening for individuals at average risk: 2020 guideline update from the American Cancer Society. CA Cancer J Clin 2020;70(5):321–46.

[15] Perkins RB, Guido RS, Castle PE, et al. 2019 ASCCP risk-based management consensus guidelines for abnormal cervical cancer screening tests and cancer precursors. J Low Genit Tract Dis 2020;24(2):102–31.

[16] Wilbur DC, Nayar R. Bethesda 2014: improving on a paradigm shift. Cytopathology 2015;26(6):339–42.

[17] Wuerthner BA, Avila-Wallace M. Cervical cancer: Screening, management, and prevention. Nurse Pract 2016;41(9):18–23.

[18] Schiffman M, Castle PE, Jeronimo J, et al. Human papillomavirus and cervical cancer. Lancet 2007;370(9590):890–907.

[19] Schiffman M, Kinney WK, Cheung LC, et al. Relative Performance of HPV and cytology components of cotesting in cervical screening. J Natl Cancer Inst 2018;110(5):501–8.

[20] Lees BF, Erickson BK, Huh WK. Cervical cancer screening: evidence behind the guidelines. Am J Obstet Gynecol 2016;214(4):438–43.

[21] Sawaya GF, Smith-McCune K. Cervical cancer screening. Obstet Gynecol 2016;127(3): 459–67.

[22] American College of Obstetricians and Gynecologists. Practice Bulletin No. 140: management of abnormal cervical cancer screening test results and cervical cancer precursors. Obstet Gynecol 2013;122(6):1338–67.

[23] American College of Obstetricians and Gynecologists. Abnormal cervical cancer screening test results 2016. Available at: https://www.acog.org/patient-resources/faqs/gynecologic-problems/abnormal-cervical-cancer-screening-test-results. Accessed June 20, 2020.

[24] Massad LS, Einstein MH, Huh WK, et al. 2012 updated consensus guidelines for the management of abnormal cervical cancer screening tests and cancer precursors. Obstet Gynecol 2013;121(4):829–46.

[25] Khan MJ, Massad LS, Kinney W, et al. A common clinical dilemma: management of abnormal vaginal cytology and human papillomavirus test results. J Low Genit Tract Dis 2016;20(2):119–25.

[26] Khan MJ, Werner CL, Darragh TM, et al. ASCCP colposcopy standards: role of colposcopy, benefits, potential harms, and terminology for colposcopic practice. J Low Genit Tract Dis 2017;21(4):223–9.

[27] Grubman J, Meinhardt S, Nambiar A, et al. Specimen fragmentation and loop electrosurgical excision procedure and cold knife cone biopsy outcomes. J Low Genit Tract Dis 2020;24(1):27–33.

[28] Maza M, Figueroa R, Bari L, et al. Effects of maintenance on quality of performance of cryotherapy devices for treatment of precancerous cervical lesions. J Low Genit Tract Dis 2018;22(1):47–51.

[29] World Health Organization (WHO). Cryosurgical equipment for the treatment of precancerous cervical lesions and prevention of cervical cancer: WHO technical specifications. 2012. Available at: https://www-who-int.proxy.library.vanderbilt.edu/reproductive-health/publications/cancers/9789241504560/en/. Accessed June 26, 2020.

[30] Melamed A, Margul DJ, Chen L, et al. Survival after minimally invasive radical hysterectomy for early-stage cervical cancer. N Engl J Med 2018;379(20):1905–14.

[31] Randall TC, Sauvaget C, Muwonge R, et al. Worthy of further consideration: An updated meta-analysis to address the feasibility, acceptability, safety and efficacy of thermal ablation in the treatment of cervical cancer precursor lesions. Prev Med 2019;118:81–91.

[32] Harper DM, DeMars LR. HPV vaccines – A review of the first decade. Gynecol Oncol 2017;146(1):196–204.

[33] Brisson M, Kim JJ, Canfell K, et al. Impact of HPV vaccination and cervical screening on cervical cancer elimination: a comparative modelling analysis in 78 low-income and lower-middle-income countries. Lancet 2020;395(10224):575–90.

[34] Gultekin M, Ramirez PT, Broutet N, et al. World Health Organization call for action to eliminate cervical cancer globally. Int J Gynecol Cancer 2020;30(4):426–7.

[35] Walker TY, Elam-Evans LD, Yankey D, et al. National, regional, state, and selected local area vaccination coverage among adolescents aged 13–17 years — United States, 2017. MMWR Morb Mortal Wkly Rep 2018;67:909–17.

[36] Centers for Disease Control and Prevention. Vaccines and preventable diseases: HPV vaccine recommendations. Available at: https://www.cdc.gov/vaccines/vpd/hpv/hcp/recommendations.html Atlanta, GA: US Department of Health and Human Services. Accessed June 15, 2020.

[37] Rutter CM, Kim JJ, Meester RGS, et al. Effect of time to diagnostic testing for breast, cervical, and colorectal cancer screening abnormalities on screening efficacy: a modeling study. Cancer Epidemiol Biomarkers Prev 2018;27(2):158–64.

[38] Musa J, Achenbach CJ, O'Dwyer LC, et al. Effect of cervical cancer education and provider recommendation for screening on screening rates: A systematic review and meta-analysis. PLoS One 2017;12(9):e0183924 [published correction appears in PLoS One. 2017 Dec 29;12 (12):e0190661].

[39] Clay JM, Daggy JK, Fluellen S, et al. Patient knowledge and attitudes toward cervical cancer screening after the 2012 screening guidelines. Patient Educ Couns 2019;102(3):411–5.

[40] Cipriano JJ, Scoloveno R, Kelly A. Increasing parental knowledge related to the human papillomavirus (HPV) Vaccine. J Pediatr Health Care 2018;32(1):29–35.

[41] Beavis AL, Levinson KL. Preventing Cervical Cancer in the United States: Barriers and Resolutions for HPV Vaccination. Front Oncol 2016;6:19.

Genitourinary Syndrome of Menopause: Screening and Treatment

Queen Henry-Okafor, PhD, FNP-BC, PMHNP-BC*,
Erin DeBruyn, DNP, APRN, WHNP-BC,
Melissa Ott, DNP, PMHNP-BC, FNP-BC,
Ginny Moore, DNP, WHNP-BC

Vanderbilt University School of Nursing, 461 21st Avenue South, Nashville, TN 37240, USA

Keywords

- Genitourinary syndrome of menopause • Hypoestrogenism • Atrophic vaginitis
- Dyspareunia • Quality of life • Menopausal hormone therapy
- Nonhormonal vaginal therapy

Key points

- Genitourinary syndrome of menopause (GSM) is a clinical state caused by reduced levels of endogenous estrogen resulting in a wide range of symptoms, including vaginal atrophy, dryness, dyspareunia, and urinary incontinence.
- GSM affects nearly 15% of premenopausal women and more than 50% of menopausal women in the United States.
- Poor quality of life in women with GSM is largely due to underdiagnosis, mainly due to stigma related to sexual dysfunction coupled with health care provider oversight.
- Individually tailored therapy using available pharmacologic and non-pharmacologic therapies can help ameliorate the syndrome.

Menopause is the phase of life after cessation of menstruation has occurred for 12 consecutive months. It is a natural process that results from normal aging of the ovaries with a subsequent decline in circulating hormones, particularly estrogen. The period preceding menopause is known as perimenopause. Many women experiencing perimenopause may report no symptoms. Of those who do report symptoms, the most common

*Corresponding author. 461 21st Avenue South, Frist Hall 354, Nashville, TN 37204. E-mail address: queen.o.henry-okafor@vanderbilt.edu

https://doi.org/10.1016/j.yfpn.2021.01.004
2589-420X/21/© 2021 Elsevier Inc. All rights reserved.

are menstrual irregularities, vasomotor symptoms, and genitourinary syndrome of menopause (GSM), formerly known as atrophic vaginitis or vulvovaginal atrophy. GSM includes genital, sexual, and urinary symptoms. It is the only category of symptoms that may worsen if left untreated. Moreover, patients are least likely to mention these symptoms to their health care provider [1,2]. As such, it is imperative that health care providers screen for and treat GSM appropriately. This article outlines the underlying causes of GSM, identifies common symptoms, discusses screening methods, and describes treatments for GSM.

BACKGROUND

GSM is the new term that was introduced in 2014 by the International Society for the Study of Women's Sexual Health and American Menopause Society as a replacement for vulvovaginal atrophy [3]. GSM is a condition experienced by women during menopause that is associated with decreased levels of endogenous estrogen. These women experience chronic vaginal and urinary health problems that tend to worsen over the years.

GSM has a high prevalence rate of 36% to almost 90% among premenopausal and postmenopausal women [4–6]. Women generally have a higher life expectancy than men and will likely spend a third of their lives in menopause [7,8]. Signs and symptoms associated with GSM include vaginal dryness, irritation, burning, dyspareunia, dysuria, urinary incontinence, and frequent urinary tract infections [1]. Most women assume that this condition is a natural process of aging for which there is no remedy, but they are unaware that treatment exists for GSM. Others may be too embarrassed to discuss these symptoms with their health care provider [9]. Consequently, this condition goes undetected, resulting in sexual dysfunction and urinary tract problems, which negatively impact quality of life.

Causes of genitourinary syndrome of menopause

The average age of menopause in the western world is age 51 [10]. Transition into menopause often begins between ages 45 and 55. As women approach menopause, their estrogen levels decline, causing symptoms such as hot flashes. GSM is caused by hypoestrogenism during perimenopause, menopause, and postmenopausal years [1]. The decline in estrogen will lead to changes in the female genitalia, including vaginal atrophy, dryness, irritation, and burning.

Hormonal therapies and chemotherapy treatment can cause estrogen deficiency and produce symptoms of GSM [11]. Other risk factors for developing GSM include alcohol abuse, cigarette smoking, lack of exercise, lack of sexual arousal and lubrication, bilateral oophorectomy, ovarian failure, and absence of vaginal birth (Fig. 1).

Women who abuse alcohol, especially during menopause, are particularly affected. Alcohol creates changes in normal physiologic response of the endocrine system, which results in decreased luteinizing hormone and subsequent ovarian atrophy, thereby creating symptoms consistent with GSM [12].

Similarly, cigarette smoking contributes to decreased circulation and impaired reception function. Women who use nicotine products are at an increased risk for developing GSM because of decreased circulation affecting the vagina by creating dryness and pain [1,13]. Women who had ovarian failure or surgical menopause (bilateral oophorectomy, partial hysterectomy, or complete hysterectomy) are likely to experience abrupt estrogen decline [1] (see Fig. 1 for a summary of GSM risk factors).

Symptoms of genitourinary syndrome of menopause
GSM refers to a collection of symptoms that results from a deficiency of estrogen and sex hormones in women in midlife. It commonly manifests with genital, sexual, and urinary symptoms [1]. In the menstruating woman, normal estrogen level modulates cellular proliferation and maturation [14]. However, with advancing age, low-estrogen levels ensue, leading to physiologic and anatomic changes. These physiologic changes lead to reduced blood flow, diminished lubrication, and an increased vulnerability to physical irritation and trauma [15]. These changes account for associated symptoms like dryness, burning sensations, and irritation of the female genitalia. Poor vaginal lubrication during intercourse, dyspareunia, and impaired sexual function characterize the sexual symptoms of GSM, translating to reduced libido and lack of interest in sexual activity.

The urinary symptoms of GSM include urinary incontinence, urgency, frequency, and recurrent urinary tract infections. Estrogen receptors found in the trigone muscles of the bladder and in the squamous epithelium of both the proximal and the distal urethra are responsible for increased sensory threshold of the bladder as well as increases in the urethral closure pressure, which promotes continence [15]. In a low estrogen state, the process becomes dysfunctional. The intrinsic sphincteric tone of the urethra is altered, and urinary symptoms, like urgency, dysuria, and recurrent urinary tract infections, occur. Most menopausal women who experience genitourinary symptoms are unaware that the symptoms are a consequence of estrogen decline associated with menopause [4].

GENITOURINARY SYNDROME OF MENOPAUSE SCREENING
Evaluation for GSM should start with a detailed clinical history. In order to accurately assess patients for potential GSM, clinicians should inquire about the presence of burning, discomfort, and lack of moisture in the vaginal area [16]. It is equally important to assess patients for different factors that could predispose them to GSM, such as surgical menopause, biologic menopause, exercise habits, tobacco use, excessive alcohol intake, absence of sexual activity, and lack of vaginal delivery/birth, particularly in premenopausal women [1]. Patients with GSM often complain of pain during sexual intercourse, as well as frequent urinary tract infections, dysuria, and frequent urination [16]. Obtaining a full medical history is necessary to identify patients with symptoms consistent with GSM.

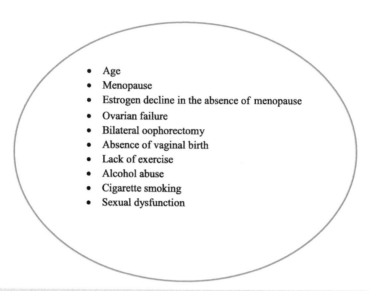

- Age
- Menopause
- Estrogen decline in the absence of menopause
- Ovarian failure
- Bilateral oophorectomy
- Absence of vaginal birth
- Lack of exercise
- Alcohol abuse
- Cigarette smoking
- Sexual dysfunction

Fig. 1. Risk factors for GSM.

Physical examination assessment of patients suspected to have GSM must include a pelvic examination. The health care provider should inspect for clitoral and labia atrophy, diminished pubic hair, decreased elasticity of the vulva, lacerations and lesions, and introital stenosis [17]. Clinicians should note that, in these women, rugae is frequently decreased, the cervix might be atrophied, cystocele and rectocele formation occasionally occur, and if there is any inflammation, it can create mild hemorrhaging of the vagina [16]. As a result, caution should be exercised in the use of the vaginal speculum, as this may cause some discomfort.

To further assist with the evaluation, the Vaginal Health Index (VHI) is a tool used to obtain a final score for defining the degree of atrophy in the genitourinary tract. VHI assigns a single score to each of the 5 parameters (vaginal elasticity, vaginal secretions, pH, the presence of petechiae on the epithelial mucous membrane, and vaginal hydration) it evaluates with the score varying between 5 and 25 [18,19]. Frequently with GSM, vaginal pH is greater than 5, as the vaginal flora begin to change during menopause [16]. Thus, the vaginal pH, pap test, and vaginal culture are useful for assessing genitourinary infection [18].

Genitourinary syndrome of menopause treatments
Nonpharmacologic
For many women, GSM can have a significant impact on sexual health and sexual practices. As mentioned earlier, women who suffer from GSM frequently experience genital symptoms (dryness, burning, and irritation) and sexual

symptoms (lack of lubrication, discomfort or pain, and impaired function). Because of these symptoms, many women are unable to continue having a fulfilling sexual life. The presence or lack of sexual activity can contribute to improving or worsening the severity of GSM. Regular sexual activity and arousal cause an increase in blood flow, oxygen, and nutrients to the vulvovaginal tissue, which helps the body to encourage the healing process naturally by keeping the tissue lubricated and elastic. Infrequent sexual activity can result in the tissue losing lubrication and elasticity and result in increased pain or discomfort. If the patient is unable to tolerate intercourse, continuing some form of arousal, like digital stimulation or oral sex, should be encouraged at least a few times per week.

The hygiene practices of patients also play a role in GSM. In order to help prevent further complications or worsening of symptoms, women should be encouraged to wear plain white, 100% cotton, brief underwear. Use of synthetic fibers and dyes in undergarments should be discouraged. Wearing a sanitary or urinary leakage pad can cause friction and irritation to the genital tissue. Women should be encouraged to use these as infrequently as possible. If women must wear a sanitary pad all the time, this indicates a need for referral to a urogynecologist. In addition to undergarments, women should be encouraged to wear loose-fitting, breathable clothing. If a woman wears activewear or sportswear clothing during exercise, they should be encouraged to remove these as soon as possible. Finally, women should be discouraged from douching, using a tub bath frequently, and using feminine washes and wipes. All these processes can eliminate the healthy vaginal flora and increase susceptibility to bacterial infections.

Nonhormonal treatments
In addition to genital stimulation and healthy hygiene practices, over-the-counter moisturizers and lubricants should be recommended. Moisturizers and lubricants provide temporary relief of vaginal dryness, burning, and irritation. Because the symptom relief is temporary, these should be considered for women with mild symptoms or in combination with another form of treatment for women with moderate to severe symptoms. Products such as Replens moisturizer and Vagisil Prohydrate are gels that can be inserted into the vagina every 2 to 3 days. If the patient does not like using a vaginal gel, another option is a hyaluronic acid vaginal insert (Revaree) that can also be used every 2 to 3 days. These products provide relief by replenishing the moisture to the epithelial cells of the vaginal walls.

Lubricants are products that are used to help lubricate the vagina for sexual purposes. These products are generally not intended to be used outside of sexual practices. There are many types of lubricants, including water soluble–based (with and without glycerin), silicone-based, oil-based (natural and synthetic), and natural (organic or vegan). Preference of type of lubricant is the patient's decision; however, the patient should be encouraged to look for a product that is similar in composition to their normal vaginal secretions.

Fractional CO_2 laser therapy (MonaLisa Touch) is another nonhormonal option. Laser therapy works by helping blood flow return to the vagina and promoting healthy tissue regeneration. This procedure is a simple procedure whereby a laser probe is placed into the vagina and activated for 5 minutes. The patient must have this procedure done for a series of treatments initially and then annually for maintenance. It is important to note that this therapy is not covered by insurance and may be cost prohibitive. Recently, the safety and efficacy of laser therapy have been called into question. In 2018, the Food and Drug Administration issued a warning regarding the safety of these devices, advising practitioners that "the safety and effectiveness of these devices for treatment of these conditions has not been established and may result in serious side effects such as vaginal scarring and burns" [20]. Table 1 summarizes nonpharmacologic treatment options.

Pharmacologic treatments
Estrogen therapy should be considered the gold standard for treatment of GSM. Systemic and vaginal estrogen may be considered after careful review of patient history to rule out contraindications, such as certain types of cancer, deep vein thrombosis, emboli, myocardial infarction, stroke, blood clotting disorders, and hepatic disorders. Systemic estrogen therapy is usually prescribed for treatment of vasomotor symptoms of menopause (hot flushes, night sweats) but also provides vaginal benefits. For women who suffer from moderate to severe symptoms of GSM, but have little to no vasomotor symptoms, localized estrogen treatment should be recommended (Table 2). Estrogen therapy treats GSM by "restoring vaginal epithelium and associated vasculature, improving vaginal secretions, lowering vaginal pH to restore healthy vaginal flora, and alleviating overall vulvovaginal symptoms" [1]. Estradiol vaginal tablets (Yuvafem, Vagifem), estradiol vaginal inserts (Imvexxy), conjugated vaginal estrogen cream (Premarin cream), estradiol vaginal cream (Estrace), and estradiol vaginal ring (ESTRING) are some of the available treatments. All these therapies work by correcting and reversing the structural changes (thinning of vaginal epithelium and atrophy of vagina, vulva, and urinary tract) owing to menopause. The recommended dosing for these localized estrogen therapies

Table 1
Examples of nonpharmacologic treatment options

Treatment	Specific therapy	Common uses
Lubricants	Water based Silicone based Oil based	Use as needed to increase comfort and pleasure during sexual activity
Moisturizers		Use daily to maintain vulvar and vaginal moisture
Self-stimulators/vibrators	Latex, nonlatex, silicone, hard plastic	Use as needed to stimulate vulvar and vaginal tissues during sexual play
Dilators	Plastic, silicone, glass	Use as needed to stretch vaginal tissues

Table 2
Examples of pharmacologic treatment options

Treatment	Product name	Initial dose	Maintenance dose
Vaginal cream	Estrace, generic	0.5–1 g/d × 2 wk	0.5–1 g 1–3 × wk
	Premarin	0.5–1 g/d × 2 wk	0.5–1 g 1–3 × wk
Vaginal inserts	Vagifem, Yuvafem	10 μg, insert 1/d × 2 wk	1 twice wk
Vaginal ring	ESTRING	2 mg releases approximately 7.5 μg/d × 90 d	Changed every 90 d
SERM	Osphena	60 mg/d	60 mg/d

is to apply to the vagina every night at bedtime for the first 14 days and then use 2 times per week for maintenance therapy. The vaginal ring is inserted into the vagina every 90 days. It is important to remember that therapeutic effects with these products are slow to appear (as little as 2 weeks for initial improvement and as long as 3–4 months for maximum improvement), and medications must be continued in order to maintain therapeutic effect. For patients who are unwilling or are unable to use a vaginal therapy, ospemifene (Osphena) is a once daily oral tablet prescribed for the treatment of moderate to severe dyspareunia. Ospemifene is a selective estrogen receptor modulator (SERM) that has estrogenic effects in the vaginal tissue, antiestrogenic effects in the breast tissue, and neutral estrogenic effects in the uterine/endometrial tissue [21]. Ospemifene may not be used with other estrogens or SERMs but may be used with over-the-counter moisturizers and lubricants (see Table 2 for examples of pharmacologic treatment options).

SUMMARY

GSM is a condition characterized by low-estrogen levels and is highly prevalent among postmenopausal women. GSM presents with the distressing symptoms of vaginal atrophy, sexual dysfunction, and urogenital infections, which negatively affect women's quality of life [1]. Despite the availability of several treatment options, this condition is still underdiagnosed and consequently undertreated [4]. A contributing factor is that most of the affected women do not seek medical help for their symptoms because of the stigma associated with having a sexual dysfunction. Health care providers should be diligent in screening all perimenopausal and postmenopausal women for signs and symptoms of GSM as well as offering personalized and tailored therapy. Appropriate screening coupled with early intervention will help mitigate the negative side effects of GSM, thus improving quality of life for perimenopausal and postmenopausal women. The authors hope that this article creates the needed awareness and motivates primary care providers into action.

CLINICS CARE POINTS

- Treatment of GSM is primarily indicated to relieve symptoms associated with diminished ovarian estrogen production.

- Distressful symptoms associated with GSM include vaginal dryness, burning, dyspareunia, dysuria urinary frequency and urethral discomfort.
- Most women with GSM do not seek care from their health care providers. As a result, clinicians should screen for these symptoms.
- First-line treatments for symptoms associated with vaginal atrophy are nonhormonal vaginal moisturizers and lubricants.
- Vaginal moisturizers should be used routinely not just during sexual activity.
- Lubricants are used only at the time of sexual activity.
- Oil-based lubricants can cause breakdown of latex condoms.
- If not contraindicated, estrogen therapy or other hormonal medications may be used as second-line treatment if first-line therapies fail to provide adequate symptom relief.
- Additionally, low-dose vaginal estrogen therapy is most effective for moderate to severe symptoms of vaginal atrophy and helps ameliorate urinary tract symptoms of GSM.
- Uncommon adverse effects of vaginal estrogen therapy include vaginal irritation, vaginal bleeding, or breast tenderness.
- Vaginal estrogen therapy should be used with caution in women with increased risk for estrogen-dependent tumors, breast, or uterine cancers.
- Vaginal estrogen therapy should be used at least 12 hours before sexual activity to avoid estrogen absorption by a sexual partner though such exposure is rarely clinically significant.
- Vaginal estrogen creams are effective for treating vaginal atrophy. Women often achieve relieve of symptoms with doses lower than the manufacturer-recommended doses.
- North American Menopause Society recommends use of low-dose vaginal estrogen therapy rather than systemic estrogen therapy for the sole treatment of symptoms of vaginal atrophy.
- Use of an opposing progestin to protect against endometrial hyperplasia or cancer is not necessary given the limited impact of low-dose estrogen on endometrial activity.
- Off-label use of vaginal testosterone can be used for concurrent treatment of low libido.
- Safety and efficacy remain a concern with use of laser or radiofrequency devices.
- Choice of therapy for management of symptoms of GSM should be guided by the individual's preference, convenience, cost, as well as systemic absorption.

Disclosure

The authors have nothing to disclose.

References

[1] Gandhi J, Chen A, Dagur G, et al. Genitourinary syndrome of menopause: an overview of clinical manifestations, pathophysiology, etiology, evaluation, and management. Am J Obstet Gynecol 2016;215(6):704–11.
[2] Goldstein I. Recognizing and treating urogenital atrophy in postmenopausal women. J Womens Health 2010;19(3):425–32.
[3] Portman DJ, Gass ML. Vulvovaginal Atrophy Terminology Consensus Conference Panel. Genitourinary syndrome of menopause: new terminology for vulvovaginal atrophy from

the International Society for the Study of Women's Sexual Health and the North American Menopause Society. Maturitas 2014;79(3):349–54.

[4] Alvisi S, Gava G, Orsili I, et al. Vaginal health in menopausal women. Medicina (Kaunas) 2019;55(10):615.

[5] DiBonaventura M, Luo X, Moffatt M, et al. The association between vulvovaginal atrophy symptoms and quality of life among postmenopausal women in the United States and Western Europe. J Womens Health 2015;24(9):713–22.

[6] Farrell AmE. Genitourinary syndrome of menopause. Aust Fam Physician 2017;46(7): 481–4.

[7] Keil K. Urogenital atrophy: diagnosis, sequelae, and management. Curr Womens Health Rep 2002;2(4):305–11.

[8] Kingsberg SA, Krychman M, Graham S, et al. The Women's EMPOWER survey: identifying women's perceptions on vulvar and vaginal atrophy and its treatment. J Sex Med 2017;14(3):413–24.

[9] Mac Bride MB, Rhodes DJ, Shuster LT. Vulvovaginal atrophy. Mayo Clin Proc 2010;85(1): 87–94.

[10] Inayat K, Danish N, Hassan L. Symptoms of menopause in peri and postmenopausal women and their attitude towards them. J Ayub Med Coll Abbottabad 2017;29(3):477–80.

[11] Faubion SS, Larkin LC, Stuenkel CA, et al. Management of genitourinary syndrome of menopause in women with or at high risk for breast cancer: consensus recommendations from The North American Menopause Society and The International Society for the Study of Women's Sexual Health. Menopause 2018;25(6):596–608.

[12] Jenczura A, Czajkowska M, Skrzypulec-Frankel A, et al. Sexual function of postmenopausal women addicted to alcohol. Int J Environ Res Public Health 2018;15(8):1639.

[13] Kagan R, Kellogg-Spadt S, Parish SJ. Practical treatment considerations in the management of genitourinary syndrome of menopause. Drugs Aging 2019;36(10):897–908.

[14] Robinson D, Cardozo L. Estrogens and the lower urinary tract. Neurourol Urodyn 2011;30(5):754–7.

[15] Robinson D, Cardozo LD. The role of estrogens in female lower urinary tract dysfunction. Urology 2003;62(4 Suppl 1):45–51.

[16] Hodges AL, Holland AC, Dehn B, et al. Diagnosis and treatment of genitourinary syndrome of menopause. Nurs Womens Health 2018;5(22):423–30.

[17] Panay N, Palacios S, Bruyniks N, et al, EVES Study investigators. Symptom severity and quality of life in the management of vulvovaginal atrophy in postmenopausal women. Maturitas 2019;124:55–61.

[18] Nappi RE, Martini E, Cucinella L, et al. Addressing vulvovaginal atrophy (VVA)/genitourinary syndrome of menopause (GSM) for healthy aging in women. Front Endocrinol 2019;10:561.

[19] Nappi RE, Particco M, Biglia N, et al. Attitudes and perceptions towards vulvar and vaginal atrophy in Italian post-menopausal women: evidence from the European REVIVE survey. Maturitas 2016;91:74–80.

[20] Food and Drug Administration. FDA warns against use of energy-based devices to perform vaginal 'rejuvenation' or vaginal cosmetic procedures: FDA safety communication. 2018. Available at: https://www.fda.gov/medical-devices/safety-communications/fda-warns-against-use-energy-based-devices-perform-vaginal-rejuvenation-or-vaginal-cosmetic. Accessed April 5, 2020.

[21] Shin JJ, Kim SK, Lee JR, et al. Ospemifene: a novel option for the treatment of vulvovaginal atrophy. J Menopausal Med 2017;23(2):79–84.

Best Practices in Breast Health and Breast Cancer Screening

Shiva Niakan, DO[a],*, Heather Love, MD, MPH[a],
Danielle Lipoff, DO, MS[b], Jesse Casaubon, DO[b],
Holly Mason, MD[b]

[a]Department of Obstetrics and Gynecology, University of Massachusetts Medical School–Baystate, 759 Chestnut Street, Springfield, MA 01199, USA; [b]Department of Surgery, University of Massachusetts Medical School–Baystate, 759 Chestnut Street, Springfield, MA 01199, USA

Keywords

• Mammography • Screening • Breast mass • Risk assessment
• Risk reducing medications

Key points

• Women commonly present to primary care providers with breast complaints.
• Primary care providers are the gateway for women to access screening.
• All women should undergo risk assessment and receive appropriate screening.
• Women considered high risk for breast cancer can benefit from enhanced surveillance or risk-reducing treatments.
• Most breast complaints, including breast masses, are benign; however, it is essential for providers to understand the evaluation and workup required to assess for malignancy.

INTRODUCTION

Breast complaints are common, and primary care providers are on the front lines of routine breast care and cancer screening [1,2]. In most cases, breast disorders are benign; however, appropriate evaluation is essential to rule out malignancy [3]. Breast cancer remains the most prevalent cancer among women; 1 in 8 women will be diagnosed in their lifetime [4].

*Corresponding author. E-mail address: Shiva.Niakan@baystatehealth.org

https://doi.org/10.1016/j.yfpn.2021.01.005
2589-420X/21/© 2021 Elsevier Inc. All rights reserved.

EVALUATION

Physical examination begins with a visual inspection of the breasts with the patient in the seated position with arms resting at the side, with observation of size, symmetry, skin changes, and assessment of nipple areolar complex. This visual inspection is followed by bilateral palpation of axillary and supraclavicular lymph nodal regions and breasts in both the upright and the supine positions. The boundaries of the breast are the inframammary fold inferiorly, the sternal border medially, and the midaxillary line laterally. Breast tissue can be located as high as the second rib, and thus, palpation should reach the clavicle to ensure that the entire breast is inspected. The breasts are evaluated in a concentric or linear pattern, systematically and consistently to encompass all breast tissue. Abnormalities are documented to include size, consistency of tissue, distance in centimeters from the nipple, and location relative to the face of a clock. The literature concerning when to start clinical breast examinations is controversial and is based on patient risk profile.

BREAST CANCER SCREENING AND RISK ASSESSMENT

Mammography is the gold standard for breast cancer screening. Professional organizations' recommendations differ regarding initiation of screening, frequency of examination, and age of discontinuation. Recommendations also vary depending on a woman's risk for developing, or personal history of, breast cancer [5]. Providers are encouraged to discuss risk factors and routine mammography with their patients, taking appropriate steps based on shared decision making.

Risk assessment

A detailed maternal and paternal family history is an essential component of every new patient evaluation to identify increased risk for inherited cancer syndromes. If a history of any cancer is identified, type of cancer and age at time of diagnosis are assessed. Although most cancers, including breast cancer, are not hereditary, identifying high-risk patients will guide screening and risk-reduction strategies. Patients with a first-degree relative with breast cancer are at increased risk for breast cancer syndromes. This risk increases with lower age at the time of diagnosis [6]. There are numerous risk assessment models, including Tyrer-Cuzick, Claus, BRCAPro, and Gail models, accessible online. No single model has been shown to be superior; studies are ongoing.

The most studied breast cancer mutations are BRCA1 and BRCA2. The BRCA genes are tumor-suppressor genes responsible for repair of DNA. The BRCA1 gene is found on chromosome 17, and BRCA2 is found on chromosome 13. The estimated risk of breast cancer in individuals with BRCA1 or BRCA2 mutations is 45% to 85% by age 70 years [7]. Despite elevated risk for breast cancer associated with these mutations, only 5% to 10% of breast cancers are due to BRCA1 or -2 mutations [8,9].

Patients with a strong family history or personal diagnosis of breast cancer may benefit from referral to genetic counseling. Women with deleterious

BRCA1/BRCA2 mutations have options for high-risk screening with chemo-prevention versus risk-reducing surgeries.

Average risk
For women at average risk, there is a 20% risk reduction from breast cancer mortality with utilization of screening mammography [10]. All organizations agree that discussions concerning screening should start at age 40. Age at which routine screening is recommended varies by society, however (Table 1) [10–13]. The age at which to stop screening varies as well. Most organizations recommend age 75 or when life expectancy is less than 10 years.

Higher-than-average risk
Women with higher-than-average risk of breast cancer may benefit from enhanced surveillance with alternating mammography and MRI. This population includes women with BRCA1 or BRCA2 mutation, women with a history of chest radiation, women with a greater than 20% lifetime risk for breast cancer, or those with a strong family history of breast cancer [5].

History of breast cancer
Women with a personal history of breast cancer are at an increased risk for breast cancer, either recurrent or a new primary. The American Society of Breast Surgeons (ASBrS) recommends annual mammography for patients over the age of 50 [14]. For patients younger than 50 or those with dense breast tissue, ASBrS recommends access to supplemental imaging in addition to routine mammography.

Oral contraceptives
Oral contraceptives (OCPs) are the most used methods of contraception. For many decades, evidence suggested increased risk for breast cancer with their use. Major landmark studies in this area are the Collaborative Group on Hormonal Factors in Breast Cancer and Nurses' Health Studies, which show a small increased risk for breast cancer in women who take OCPs [15,16]. A more recent study in the *New England Journal of Medicine* corroborated these findings, demonstrating increased risk of developing breast cancer by a factor

Table 1
Breast cancer screening recommendations

Age to start breast cancer screening for average risk women by organization		
Age 40	Age 45	Age 50
ASBrS	ACS	USPSTF
ACOG		
ACR		
NCCN		

Abbreviations: ACOG, American College of Obstetricians and Gynecologists; ACR, American College of Radiology; ACS, American Cancer Society; NCCN, National Comprehensive Cancer Network.

of 1.20 in women using OCPs [17]. It is important to note that OCPs are essential in treating dysmenorrhea and preventing undesired pregnancy. They also decrease risk of ovarian, uterine, and colon cancer [18]. For most patients, overall benefits of OCPs outweigh risks.

Hormone replacement therapy

Hormone replacement therapy (HRT) is used to mediate the symptoms of menopause, including vasomotor changes, osteoporosis, and cardiovascular disease. Its use remains controversial because of conflicting data. One major landmark study in this area is The Women's Health Initiative (WHI) from in 2002, which looked at estrogen and progesterone versus placebo in postmenopausal women and was terminated early because of a high incidence of breast cancer and cardiovascular disease in the experimental group. These findings led to rapid decline in use of HRT by clinicians. Since the initial findings of WHI, further studies evaluated the data more closely, finding that HRT may decrease coronary heart disease, decrease the risk of osteoporosis, and improve quality of life.

Currently, the Food and Drug Administration approves use of HRT only for vasomotor symptoms, and the current body of evidence continues to suggest increased risk of breast cancer with use of HRT. In the WHI, increased risk of breast cancer was noted in patients using combination therapy with estrogen and progesterone, but not in the patients using estrogen alone. The Million Women Study demonstrated increased risk for estrogen alone as well as in combination; however, the risk was higher with the combination form of HRT [19]. Other studies have found that progesterone alone does not increase the risk of breast cancer [20]. A more recent study examined 2 trials from the WHI and found that women who had undergone a hysterectomy and taking estrogen alone were found to have a decreased risk of breast cancer. The study again demonstrated increased risk of breast cancer in postmenopausal women taking combination therapy [21]. HRT does have significant benefits that cannot be discounted; use of HRT should be individualized with shared decision making.

Clinical breast examinations

Evidence does not clearly demonstrate that either self-breast examinations or clinical examinations by a provider improve breast cancer outcomes. The US Preventive Services Task Force (USPSTF) recommends against teaching breast self-examination [13]; however, some studies suggest that approximately 50% of breast cancer in women older than 50 years may be detected by self-examination. Thus, most organizations recommend breast awareness and encourage women to seek care if they note changes in their breast [13].

Risk-reducing medication

The USPSTF recommends risk-reducing agents, such as tamoxifen, raloxifene, or aromatase inhibitors, for women at increased risk of breast cancer, including women over the age of 35 with atypical hyperplasia or lobular carcinoma in situ [22]. Tamoxifen and raloxifene are selective estrogen receptor modulators that inhibit estrogen receptors in the breast and therefore prohibit proliferation. Aromatase inhibitors stop the conversion of androgens to estrogen, which decreases the overall estrogen available in the body, and ultimately also inhibits proliferation of estrogen-sensitive cells, decreasing the risk of breast cancer development.

The USPSTF evaluated 10 different trials and found a moderate benefit of tamoxifen, with a decrease in risk of estrogen-positive breast cancer in postmenopausal women at high risk for breast cancer. One study evaluating tamoxifen found a nearly 50% decrease in breast cancer risk [23]. Most studies implemented risk-reducing medications for 3 to 5 years and demonstrated persistent benefits for up to 8 years after discontinuation [24]. However, despite recommendations from USPSTF and American Cancer Society and other strong evidence, this is not a highly used practice. In 1 study, only 10% to 30% of primary care providers report ever prescribing these medications for prevention of breast cancer [25]. Because of the complexity regarding decision making for the use of risk-reducing medications, it is reasonable to refer these patients to a high-risk breast cancer program for consultation.

SCREENING AND DIAGNOSTIC IMAGING
Breast Imaging Reporting and Data System
The Breast Imaging Reporting and Data System (BI-RADS) is a numerical score (0–6) developed by the American College of Radiology to standardize the reporting of breast imaging and recommendations for management (Table 2) [26].

Mammography
Since the introduction of film mammography in the late 1970s, breast cancer death rates declined because early detection results in more effective management [3]. The sensitivity of mammography correlates inversely to the density of breast tissue [13]. Alternative imaging modalities improve detection. These imaging modalities include digital mammography and digital breast

Table 2			
Breast Imaging Reporting and Data System assessment categories			
	Definition	Management	Risk of cancer, %
BI-RADS 0	Incomplete assessment	Additional imaging	—
BI-RADS 1	Negative examination	Routine screening	~0
BI-RADS 2	Benign findings	Routine screening	~0
BI-RADS 3	Probably benign findings	Short-term follow-up	<2
BI-RADS 4	Suspicious abnormality	Biopsy	2–95
BI-RADS 5	Highly suggestive of malignancy	Biopsy	>95
BI-RADS 6	Biopsy-proven malignancy		

tomosynthesis (DBT or 3-dimensional mammography), which uses multiple images and angles to improve assessment. The additional images limit artifacts caused by superimposition of dense breast tissue. DBT has higher sensitivity, improved detection rates, and decreased false positive rates, especially in patients with dense breast tissue [27,28]. It is increasingly available; however, not all insurances cover the additional cost.

Ultrasound

Breast ultrasound (US) uses sound waves to create a digital image of the breast tissue.

Recommendations for use, according to American College of Radiology and ASBrS, are as follows [12,14]:

- Screening women at increased risk for breast cancer in addition to mammography
- An adjunct to mammography for women with extremely dense breast tissue
- Evaluation of a palpable mass
  - Primary imaging tool in women under the age of 30
  - In conjunction with diagnostic mammography for any palpable mass in women over the age of 30

BREAST MRI

Contrast-enhanced breast MRI is more sensitive than mammography or US in the detection of breast cancer [29]. Screening breast MRI is indicated for high-risk patients. Higher sensitivity for detection of malignant lesions increases false positive rate, identifying lesions that appear suspicious on imaging, but are later found to be benign on biopsy. MRI is also costly as compared with US and mammography.

BREAST BIOPSY

For suspicious lesions detected by physical examination or imaging, percutaneous biopsy is recommended for diagnosis. Together, physical examination, imaging, and biopsy constitute the "triple test." When concordant, the triple test is greater than 99% accurate [30]. When malignancy is suggested by any one of these tests or there is discordance, excision is indicated [31].

COMMON BREAST CONCERNS

Mastalgia

Mastalgia, or breast pain, is a common complaint and accounts for most breast-related visits. Although mastalgia causes concern for malignancy among patients, breast cancer is rarely found in the absence of other clinical findings [4]. Mastalgia may be cyclical, noncyclical, or extramammary [32] and may interfere with sexual or physical activity [33].

Cyclical pain is secondary to normal hormonal changes associated with menses or exogenous sex hormones associated with contraception, ovulation induction, or management of abnormal bleeding. Patients with breast pain are more likely to seek medical attention, receive mammography under the age of 35, and undergo biopsy than asymptomatic patients [33]. It may also result in increased anxiety and depression [34]. General considerations for treatment of mastalgia are to wear supportive bras, take over-the-counter analgesics such as ibuprofen or acetaminophen, and to decrease one's caffeine intake.

Noncyclic pain accounts for one-third of mastalgia. Causes include trauma, thrombophlebitis, lactational concerns including obstructed ducts and mastitis, cysts, and more rarely, tumors and rapidly enlarging cancers [32]. This type of pain is more common in postmenopausal women and tends to be unilateral. It is more often related to anatomic cause than hormonal. It rarely indicates underlying malignancy [35].

Nipple discharge

Another common and frequently benign problem is nipple discharge. Detailed history and physical examination can usually determine an accurate diagnosis. If a palpable mass or abnormality on imaging is identified in conjunction with nipple discharge, independent evaluation of these findings is indicated [36].

When discharge is bilateral, present only with manual expression, originating from multiple ducts, and green or milky in color, it is most likely a physiologic cause [4]. Milky discharge is common and normal during pregnancy and lactation and may persist for up to 1 year postpartum or following weaning of infants. Occasionally, women may experience frankly bloody discharge at onset of lactation, which should resolve within 1 to 2 weeks. Further evaluation is indicated if it persists or is unilateral [4].

Galactorrhea or bilateral milky discharge outside of the peripartum period is often due to an extrinsic cause, such as an endocrinopathy or medication side effects. Evaluation should include medical and surgical history, medications, reproductive history, skin, and gastrointestinal symptoms. It is important to evaluate thyroid function as well as prolactin levels. Neurologic features, including headache and visual field defects, may be due to the mass effect of a potential pituitary microadenoma [36]. Normal physiologic processes, including stress, eating, sleep, orgasm, breast stimulation, exercise, late follicular and early luteal phases of menstruation, and pregnancy, may increase serum prolactin levels, causing galactorrhea. Prolactin levels may also be increased secondary to failure of regulatory mechanisms, including pituitary adenomas and hypothyroidism [36]. A normal prolactin level can narrow the differential diagnosis and therefore is useful in the workup of these patients.

There are medical and surgical conditions as well as medications that can can elevate prolactin levels. These are listed in Table 3 and 4 [37].

Medications that may increase prolactin levels are listed in Table 4 [37].

Suspicious discharge is more frequently unilateral, uniductal, spontaneous, and clear, serous, or bloody in nature [4]. Discharge is more concerning in the presence of a mass or abnormality on imaging. Causes include ductal ectasia, fibrocystic breast changes, intraductal papilloma, intraductal carcinoma, and invasive ductal carcinoma.

Table 3
Medical and surgical conditions that may increase prolactin levels

• Chronic renal failure	• Growth hormone–	• Herpes zoster
• Hypothyroidism	producing pituitary lesions	• Hypernephroma
• Hypothalamic lesions	• Prior thoracotomy or thoracic neoplasm	

Bloody nipple discharge is most commonly a result of an intraductal papilloma. These lesions are not precursors to cancer but may be considered a marker of elevated lifetime risk for carcinoma. They may also include areas of atypia or ductal carcinoma in situ, and if this is identified on core needle biopsy, subsequent excision is warranted [38].

In women with nipple discharge, it is important to rule out pregnancy and to assess for breast masses, which if present will require further workup. For women younger than 30 years of age, retroareolar breast US is the imaging method of choice. For women over the age of 30, breast US and possibly mammography may be considered. Although imaging is usually of low yield, it may be considered in the workup for nipple discharge [39].

Mastitis

Mastitis may be lactational or nonlactational. Peripartum mastitis is most common in the first 3 months of lactation and presents with erythema, pain, fever, and malaise. It occurs through a process of nipple trauma, poor milk drainage, or engorgement secondary to swelling and compression of milk ducts. It occurs in 2% to 10% of lactating women, and those with a history of prior infection remain at higher risk [40]. The most common organisms include *Staphylococcus aureus*, methicillin-resistant *S aureus*, and less frequently, *Streptococcus pyogenes* (group A or B), *Escherichia coli*, *Bacteroides* species, *Corynebacterium* species, and coagulase-negative staphylococci.

Management includes frequent and complete emptying of the breast, warm compresses, and empiric antibiotics, such as dicloxacillin, cephalexin, or erythromycin or clindamycin. If no clinical improvement, US is indicated to assess for underlying abscess that may necessitate needle aspiration or incision and drainage.

Table 4
Medications that may elevate prolactin levels

Neuroleptics	Antidepressants	Antihypertensives	Gastrointestinal	Other drugs
• Phenothiazine	• Tricyclic and	• Verapamil	• Metoclopramide	• Opiates
• Thioxanthenes	tetracyclics	• Methyldopa	• Domperidone	• Estrogen
• Butyrophenones	• Monoamine	• Reserpine	• Histamine	• Protease
• Atypical	oxidase inhibitors		receptor blockers	inhibitors
antipsychotics	• Selective serotonin			• Cocaine
	reuptake inhibitors			

Nonlactational mastitis describes inflammation of the breast that may or may not be a result of microbial infection and thus may not resolve with antibiotic therapy [4]. Types of nonlactational mastitis include periductal mastitis, idiopathic granulomatous mastitis [41], and the extremely uncommon tuberculous mastitis [42].

Dermatologic concerns

Common dermatologic problems of the breast include psoriasis, eczema, and contact dermatitis. These dermatologic problems may be treated as they would be elsewhere on the body [4]. Patients may develop hidradenitis suppurativa in the axilla and infections with *Candida albicans* along the inframammary folds. These infections can also occur as nipple thrush in lactating women.

Dermatologic changes may also be an indication of underlying malignancy. Paget disease is a rare cancer of the nipple and areola frequently associated with an underlying area of ductal carcinoma in situ. Common presentation is scaly, ulcerated, eczematous changes of the nipple, which can also be associated with nipple discharge [43,44]. A wedge or skin punch biopsy is recommended to confirm diagnosis. Diagnostic imaging with mammography to rule out underlying cancer is also recommended.

Skin changes are noted in cases of inflammatory breast cancer, including erythema or skin edema with the classic "peau d'orange" appearance. Inflammatory breast cancer may not present as a discrete palpable mass and should be suspected in patients with suspected mastitis that does not respond to antibiotic therapy.

Benign breast mass

Benign breast masses are more common in the second decade of life, peaking in the fourth to fifth decades Table 5. Clinical features of benign masses and breast cancer may overlap significantly, and some benign breast disease may indicate a predisposition for malignancy [4]. Once a diagnosis of benign disease is established with use of imaging and percutaneous needle biopsy (Fig. 1), it may generally be treated with symptomatic relief and reassurance [45].

Benign breast disorders may be histologically divided into categories of nonproliferative, proliferative without atypia, and atypical hyperplasia [45]. The categories are used to predict the aggregate risk of future breast cancer.

Nonproliferative breast lesions include simple cysts, mild hyperplasia, and papillary apocrine change. Simple cysts are most common and found in one-third of women aged 35 to 50 years [45]. They vary in size from microscopic to palpable and may be found incidentally or on physical examination. Simple cysts lack internal septations or mural thickening and confer no increased risk of cancer. They may be managed expectantly or drained if bothersome to the patient [46]. Complicated cysts demonstrated internal echoes on sonography and may show similar characteristics as solid masses. Aspiration may assist in diagnosis. Complex cysts contain septa or intracystic masses and may be the initial presentation of papilloma or carcinoma; thus, biopsy is recommended [47].

Table 5
Common breast pathologic conditions

Benign complaints	Benign masses	Cancer
• Nipple discharge	• Simple cyst	• Invasive breast cancer
• Mastalgia	• Fibroadenoma	• Paget disease
• Mastitis	• Intraductal papilloma	• Phyllodes tumor
• Dermatologic concerns	• Hyperplasia	• Ductal carcinoma in situ
	• Papillary apocrine change	
	High risk for cancer	
	• Atypical ductal hyperplasia	
	• Lobular carcinoma in situ	

Proliferative breast lesions without atypia include fibroadenoma, intraductal papilloma, moderate hyperplasia, sclerosing adenosis, and radial scar. Fibroadenoma is the most common proliferative lesion in adolescent girls and women 25 years of age or younger. Fibroadenomas tend to involute in menopause, but account for approximately 12% of masses in this population. Fibroadenomas represent a focal developmental abnormality, and the majority may be followed without excision. A rapidly growing fibroadenoma merits excision, as it may be clinically indistinguishable from a phyllodes tumor [48].

Moderate hyperplasia involves the epithelial cell layers of multiple ducts without atypia and is associated with a small to moderate increased risk of future breast cancer development. It does not warrant excision.

Atypical ductal hyperplasia is associated with a 4-fold risk of invasive cancer [45]. Surgical excision is recommended to rule out malignancy in the area of atypia itself. Patients with atypical ductal hyperplasia should be considered high risk, monitored appropriately, and considered for risk-reducing medication.

BREAST CANCER

Early detection of breast cancer and an improved understanding of the biology of breast cancer have allowed for dramatic changes in treatment strategies. In

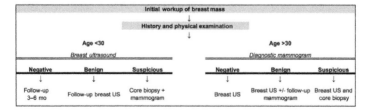

Fig. 1. Evaluation of breast mass.

addition to assessing estrogen and progesterone receptor status, the Her-2 growth factor is now routinely tested. The presence of estrogen and/or progesterone receptors allows for endocrine therapy (tamoxifen, aromatase inhibitors, ovarian suppression). The presence of Her-2, although a sign of aggressiveness, can be targeted with monoclonal antibody treatment (trastuzumab, pertuzumab). Molecular profiling of hormone receptor–positive tumors can indicate whether there is benefit to chemotherapy in addition to endocrine therapy, which has dramatically altered the indications for adjuvant cytotoxic chemotherapy. There has also been a deescalation in surgical treatment of breast cancer, especially those over the age of 70 with hormone receptor–positive breast cancer, for whom removal of lymph nodes and/or breast radiation may not be necessary. Put together, women faced with a diagnosis of breast cancer have more options with proven benefit than in previous years with treatment directed at their particular cancer.

SUMMARY

Breast-related complaints are a common reason for presentation for evaluation in the health care setting. Although most breast disorders are benign, an understanding of examination findings and methods of evaluation is essential.

Disclosure

The authors of this article have no financial interests to disclose.

References

[1] Pearlman MD, Griffin JL. Benign breast disease. Obstet Gynecol 2010;116(3):747–58.
[2] Price DW, Xu S, McClure D. Effect of CME on primary care and OB/GYN treatment of breast masses. J Contin Educ Health Prof 2005;25(4):240–7.
[3] Klein S. Evaluation of palpable breast masses. Am Fam Physician 2005;71(9):1731–8.
[4] American Cancer Society. Cancer Facts & Figures, 2017. Atlanta, GA: American Cancer Society; 2017.
[5] Bevers TB, Helvie M, Bonaccio E, et al. Breast cancer screening and diagnosis, version 3.2018, NCCN clinical practice guidelines in oncology. J Natl Compr Cancer Netw 2018;16(11):1362–89.
[6] McPherson KM, Steel CM, Dixon JM. APC of breast diseases: breast cancer - epidemiology, risk factors, and genetics. BMJ 1994;309:1003.
[7] King MC, Marks JH, Mandell JB. Breast and ovarian cancer risks due to inherited mutations in BRCA1 and BRCA2. New York Breast Cancer Study Group. Science 2003;302:643–6.
[8] Peto J, Collins N, Barfoot R, et al. Prevalence of BRCA1 and BRCA2 gene mutations in patients with early-onset breast cancer. J Natl Cancer Inst 1999;91(11):943–9.
[9] Antoniou AC, Pharoah PD, McMullan G, et al. A comprehensive model for familial breast cancer incorporating BRCA1, BRCA2 and other genes. Br J Cancer 2002;86(1):76–83.
[10] Oeffinger KC, Fontham ETH, Etzioni R, et al. Breast cancer screening for women at average risk: 2015 guideline update from the American Cancer Society. JAMA 2015;314(15): 1599–614.
[11] American College of Obstetricians-Gynecologists. Practice bulletin no. 122: breast cancer screening. Obstet Gynecol 2011;118(2 Pt 1):372–82.
[12] Lee CH, Dershaw DD, Kopans D, et al. Breast cancer screening with imaging: recommendations from the Society of Breast Imaging and the ACR on the use of mammography, breast MRI, breast ultrasound, and other technologies for the detection of clinically occult breast cancer. J Am Coll Radiol 2010;7(1):18–27.

[13] Siu AL. U.S. Preventive Services Task Force. Screening for breast cancer: U.S. Preventive Services Task Force Recommendation Statement [published correction appears in Ann Intern Med. 2016 Mar 15;164(6):448]. Ann Intern Med 2016;164(4):279–96.

[14] American Society of Breast Surgeons Position Statement on screening mammography. 2019. Available at: https://www.breastsurgeons.org/. Accessed June 28, 2020.

[15] Hunter DJ, Colditz GA, Hankinson SE, et al. Oral contraceptive use and breast cancer: a prospective study of young women. Cancer Epidemiol Biomarkers Prev 2010;19: 2496–502.

[16] Breast cancer and hormonal contraceptives: further results. Collaborative Group on Hormonal Factors in Breast Cancer. Contraception 1996;54(3 Suppl):1S–106S.

[17] Mørch LS, Skovlund CW, Hannaford PC, et al. Contemporary hormonal contraception and the risk of breast cancer. N Engl J Med 2017;377:2228–39.

[18] Iversen L, Sivasubramaniam S, Lee AJ, et al. Lifetime cancer risk and combined oral contraceptives: the Royal College of General Practitioners' Oral Contraception Study. Am J Obstet Gynecol 2017;216(6):580.e9.

[19] The Million Women Study: design and characteristics of the study population. The Million Women Study Collaborative Group. Breast Cancer Res 1999;1(1):73–80.

[20] Samson M, Porter N, Orekoya O, et al. Progestin and breast cancer risk: a systematic review. Breast Cancer Res Treat 2016;155(1):3–12.

[21] Chlebowski RT, Rohan TE, Manson JE, et al. Breast cancer after use of estrogen plus progestin and estrogen alone: analyses of data from 2 Women's Health Initiative randomized clinical trials. JAMA Oncol 2015;1(3):296-305.

[22] US Preventive Services Task Force, Owens DK, Davidson KW, et al. Medication use to reduce risk of breast cancer: US Preventive Services Task Force Recommendation Statement. JAMA 2019;322(9):857–67.

[23] Fisher B, Costantino JP, Wickerham DL, et al. Tamoxifen for prevention of breast cancer: report of the National Surgical Adjuvant Breast and Bowel Project P-1 Study. J Natl Cancer Inst 1998;90(18):1371–88.

[24] Nelson HD, Fu R, Zakher B, et al. Medication use for the risk reduction of primary breast cancer in women: updated evidence report and systematic review for the US Preventive Services Task Force. JAMA 2019;322(9):868–86.

[25] Kaplan CP, Haas JS, Pérez-Stable EJ, et al. Factors affecting breast cancer risk reduction practices among California physicians. Prev Med 2005;41(1):7–15.

[26] Balleyguier C, Ayadi S, Van Nguyen K, et al. BIRADS classification in mammography. Eur J Radiol 2007;61(2):192–4.

[27] Rafferty EA, Park JM, Philpotts LE, et al. Assessing radiologist performance using combined digital mammography and breast tomosynthesis compared with digital mammography alone: results of a multicenter, multireader trial. Radiology 2013;266:104–13.

[28] Zuley ML, Bandos AI, Ganott MA, et al. Digital breast tomosynthesis versus supplemental diagnostic mammographic views for evaluation of noncalcified breast lesions. Radiology 2013;266:89–95.

[29] Kuhl CK, Schrading S, Leutner CC, et al. Mammography, breast ultrasound, and magnetic resonance imaging for surveillance of women at high familial risk for breast cancer. J Clin Oncol 2005;23(33):8469–76.

[30] Morris KT, Pommier RF, Morris A, et al. Usefulness of the triple test score for palpable breast masses. Arch Surg 2001;136:1008–12.

[31] Wai CJ, Al-Mubarak G, Homer MJ, et al. A modified triple test for palpable breast masses: the value of ultrasound and core needle biopsy. Ann Surg Oncol 2013;20(3):850–5.

[32] Smith RL, Pruthi S, Fitzpatrick LA. Evaluation and management of breast pain. Mayo Clin Proc 2004;79(3):353–72.

[33] Ader DN, Browne MW. Prevalence and impact of cyclic mastalgia in a United States clinic-based sample. Am J Obstet Gynecol 1997;177(1):126–32.

[34] Downey HM, Deadman JM, Davis C, et al. Psychological characteristics of women with cyclical mastalgia. Breast Dis 1993;6:99–105.

[35] Lumachi F, Ermani M, Brandes AA, et al. Breast complaints and risk of breast cancer. Population-based study of 2,879 self-selected women and long-term follow-up. Biomed Pharmacother 2002;56(2):88–92.

[36] Falkenberry SS. Nipple discharge. Obstet Gynecol Clin North Am 2002;29(1):21–9.

[37] Molitch ME. Medication-induced hyperprolactinemia. Mayo Clin Proc 2005;80(8): 1050–7.

[38] Wen X, Cheng W. Nonmalignant breast papillary lesions at core-needle biopsy: a meta-analysis of underestimation and influencing factors. Ann Surg Oncol 2013;20(1):94–101.

[39] Salzman B, Collins E, Hersh L. Common breast problems. Am Fam Physician 2019;99(8): 505–14.

[40] Committee on Health Care for Underserved Women, American College of Obstetricians and Gynecologists. ACOG Committee Opinion No. 361: breastfeeding: maternal and infant aspects. Obstet Gynecol 2007;109(2 Pt 1):479–80.

[41] Dixon JM, Ravisekar O, Chetty U, et al. Periductal mastitis and duct ectasia: different conditions with different aetiologies. Br J Surg 1996;83(6):820–2.

[42] Farrokh D, Alamdaran A, Feyzi Laeen A, et al. Tuberculous mastitis: a review of 32 cases. Int J Infect Dis 2019;87:135–42.

[43] Chen CY, Sun LM, Anderson BO. Paget disease of the breast: changing patterns of incidence, clinical presentation, and treatment in the U.S. Cancer 2006;107(7):1448–58.

[44] Caliskan M, Gatti G, Sosnovskikh I, et al. Paget's disease of the breast: the experience of the European Institute of Oncology and review of the literature. Breast Cancer Res Treat 2008;112(3):513–21.

[45] Rungruang B, Kelley JL 3rd. Benign breast diseases: epidemiology, evaluation, and management. Clin Obstet Gynecol 2011;54(1):110–24.

[46] Guray M, Sahin AA. Benign breast diseases: classification, diagnosis, and management. Oncologist 2006;11(5):435–49.

[47] Tea MK, Grimm C, Fink-Retter A, et al. The validity of complex breast cysts after surgery. Am J Surg 2009;197(2):199–202.

[48] Marcil G, Wong S, Trabulsi N, et al. Fibroepithelial breast lesions diagnosed by core needle biopsy demonstrate a moderate rate of upstaging to phyllodes tumors. Am J Surg 2017;214(2):318–22.

Smoking and Maternal Health
Evidence that Female Infertility Can Be Attributed to Smoking and Improved with Smoking Cessation

Julia M. Steed, PhD, APRN, FNP-BC, CTTS[a],*,
Shaunna Parker, APRN, WHNP-BC[b], Breia Reed, MS[c]

[a]Vanderbilt University School of Nursing, 461 21st Avenue, Frist Hall 358, Nashville, TN 37204, USA; [b]Vanderbilt University School of Nursing, 461 21st Avenue, 603A Godchaux Hall, Nashville, TN 37204, USA; [c]Meharry Medical School, 1005 Dr DB Todd Jr Boulevard, Nashville, TN 37208, USA

Keywords

- Infertility • Female • Smoking • Tobacco use disorder • Smoking cessation
- Reproduction

Key points

- Infertility among female smokers is twice the rate of infertility found in non-smokers, yet many primary care providers are unaware that smoking causes a significant decrease in fertility.
- Infertility caused by tobacco use disorder can be managed successfully in a primary care setting and resolved within a year or less of abstinence.
- A highly effective, but simple management approach to treat tobacco dependence among reproductive-aged women includes brief, individualized counseling, referral to a stop smoking program, and support via routine follow-up.
- The reversible dose-dependent relationship between smoking and infertility is an important research finding that can be a powerful incentive to quit for infertile women who smoke.

INTRODUCTION

Medical visits for female infertility have increased over the last 10 years owing to a shift in social norms now that 20% of women have their first child after 35 years of age and the wide spread accessibility of effective treatment options

*Corresponding author. E-mail address: julia.m.steed@vanderbilt.edu

https://doi.org/10.1016/j.yfpn.2021.01.006
2589-420X/21/© 2021 Elsevier Inc. All rights reserved.

[1]. Primary care providers can often treat cases of infertility owing to the general nature of the cause in some cases. The most significant risk factors that impact female infertility include both nonmodifiable and modifiable risk factors, which include age, substance abuse, abnormal weight, stress, and environmental factors. Owing to age, a nonmodifiable risk factor, a woman has half the chance of becoming pregnant at 35 years of age compared with when she was 25 years old. The quality and quantity of a woman's eggs begin to decrease with increasing age with decreasing rates that range from 7.3% to 9.1% in women aged 15 to 34 years, 25% in women ages 35 to 39 years old, and 30% in women aged 40 to 44 years [2,3]. Conversely, cigarette smoking is a modifiable risk factor for female infertility. Infertility among female smokers of reproductive age is twice the rate of infertility found in nonsmokers, and female smokers must often attempt twice as many in vitro fertilization cycles to achieve pregnancy than a nonsmoker [4]. Tobacco use disorder among female smokers can be effectively managed and treated within the scope of primary care.

As the leading cause of preventable death in the United States, cigarette smoking harms nearly every organ in the body and is known to cause damage to the cervix and fallopian tubes [5]. Approximately 21% of reproductive age women (15–49 year old) in the United States smoke cigarettes [6]. Although the negative effects of tobacco use disorder and cigarette smoking on female fertility have become apparent in the reproductive health literature, these risks are not generally appreciated among the medical or lay public [4]. It is imperative that primary care providers understand how cigarette smoking may decrease fertility by harming the reproductive system and know how to manage a smoking cessation treatment plan for the infertile female smoker. This knowledge can then be used to guide preconception counseling about smoking cessation efforts among reproductive-aged women and those already diagnosed with infertility. This article focuses on the evaluation, management, and treatment implications of smoking on female infertility in a primary care setting.

REPRODUCTIVE CONSEQUENCES OF SMOKING CIGARETTES

The mechanisms associated with female infertility have not been elucidated completely, although a select few of the more than 700 toxic chemicals found in cigarette smoke have been scientifically investigated and found to contribute to reproductive toxicity [7]. For example, nicotine, carbon monoxide, and cyanide cause vasoconstriction and cell growth retardation, which may lead to placental insufficiency, embryonic and fetal growth restriction, and eventual fetal demise [8]. Moreover, cadmium, a known heavy metal that is toxic to the ovaries, was found in higher concentrations in the follicular fluid of smokers than nonsmokers, along with lipid peroxidation, a marker of intrafollicular oxidative stress [9,10].

Further evidence suggests that there are negative effects of cigarette smoking in relation to treatment for infertility. For example, active smoking was found to interfere with successful ovulation induction for women with polycystic ovary syndrome, and active smoking among couples was associated with decreased effectiveness of egg production with infertility treatments using estrogen modulators [11]. The identified associations were independent of effects related to age, body mass index (BMI), sperm concentration, intercourse frequency, and study drug randomization [11,12]. Each year a woman smoked was associated with a 9% increase in the risk of an unsuccessful infertility treatment using assisted reproductive technology (95% confidence interval [CI], 1.0–1.16; $P<.02$) [13]. Even comparatively low levels of tobacco and nicotine can have a significant impact on a woman's fertility. One study reported that a woman who has ever smoked during her lifetime and was undergoing assisted reproductive technology was more likely to fail to conceive (relative risk [RR], 2.71; 95% CI, 1.37–5.35; $P<.01$) or achieve a live birth (RR, 2.51; 95% CI, 1.11–5.67; $P<.03$) when compared with a nonsmoker [13]. Another study reported that success of in vitro fertilization can be decreased by as much as 50% among female smokers compared with women undergoing in vitro fertilization who have never smoked [14].

Published systematic literature reviews and large-scale population-based studies have verified estimates of smoking's effects on female infertility, independent of other risk factors, and the results are unlikely to have occurred by chance [8,15]. One study found that active smoking was significantly associated with a failure to conceive within 1 year, and that the percentage of women experiencing conception delay for more than 1 year was 54% higher for smokers than in nonsmokers [8]. Other studies supported these findings by identifying that smoking was associated with several dysfunctional reproductive effects that can result in female infertility, such as a shorter menstrual cycle length (24 days), accelerated follicular depletion, and an earlier age of menopause [8]. There is also evidence that the effects on fertility were seen only in women smoking more than 20 cigarettes per day (1 pack per day) or an increasing delay to conception was found to correlate with increasing daily numbers of cigarettes smoked [8,16]. However, a trend for active smoking was identified regardless of the frequency of consumption as well [10,16].

HISTORY
Female infertility
An evaluation for female infertility in the primary care setting should be initiated with a comprehensive history to include questions that may identify potential causes of dysfunction of the female reproductive system, including endocrinology and immunologic conditions [17]. Historical factors concerning the patient's duration of infertility/previous treatment, pattern of menstrual cycles, history of sexual dysfunction, use of lubricant or vaginal douches after sex that may contain a spermicide, personal and family medical and reproductive history, obstetric and contraceptive history, previous screening for genetic issues, and a history of venous thrombotic events should be elicited from the patient at a minimum to investigate the issue [17,18]. In addition, the patient's

social and lifestyle history should be solicited to assess use of cigarettes, alcohol, or illicit drugs; hazards associated with their occupation; and lifestyle management of health status (eg, exercise and diet) [17].

Smoking status

Documentation of smoking status should indicate the following:

1. Whether the individual is an active, former smoker, or never smoker.
2. Whether the individual is a daily or nondaily smoker.
3. Frequency of cigarette consumption based on packs per day.
4. Whether the individual is a "light" or "heavy" smoker.
5. Lifetime smoking history (pack-years).

An active smoking status is defined as a self-report of current or recent exposure to inhaled nicotine from tobacco through a cigarette within the past month (30-day point prevalence) [19]. This definition applies to both daily and nondaily cigarette smokers, but excludes ingestion of other tobacco products, such as cigars, pipes, and smokeless tobacco in which nicotine is absorbed in the oral or nasal cavity [20]. The definition also excludes inhaling nicotine from an electronic nicotine device system, commonly referred to as e-cigarettes or vapes. Smoking status is also assessed by evaluating the prevalence of current cigarette consumption (daily or nondaily) along with the frequency of consumption (number of cigarettes smoked per day) [7]. Current smoking frequency and consumption rates may significantly impact medication decisions when treating tobacco dependence. For example, a "heavy" smoker may develop nicotine tolerance and begin to exhibit withdrawal symptoms anytime nicotine is absent, even overnight [2,21]. If possible, a lifetime smoking history, or pack-years, is valuable to obtain; it is a calculation of the patient's current smoking prevalence and frequency and the number of years smoked for each change in prevalence or frequency.

Additional historical factors to inquire to comprehensively assess smoking history include questions to evaluate at what age smoking was initiated, regular or menthol cigarette use, other concomitant use of other tobacco products (e-cigarette, smokeless tobacco, hookah, etc.), a general psychosocial history (working status, exposure to cohabitants who smoke, quality of support systems/spiritual life, etc), a mental health history, and experience with quitting or a quit attempt(s). A subjective history to obtain details about attempts to quit smoking in the past can be facilitated by asking the woman to describe the longest period they voluntarily went without smoking. If there were multiple, discrete attempts made to quit smoking, providers are encouraged to gather as much information about each attempt, specifically regarding prescription and over-the-counter medication use and tolerance. A previous history of depression, use of antidepressants in the past, and onset of depression during previous attempts to quit smoking should also be obtained. Barriers to smoking cessation include childhood or teenage smoking initiation, menthol cigarette use, high nicotine dependence, living with a disability, exposure to cigarette smoking in the household, high stress levels, poor social support, and a psychiatric comorbidity [7,22]. Factors associated with higher smoking cessation and abstinence rates include high motivation to quit and readiness to change smoking behaviors, moderate to high self-efficacy, and supportive social networks [7].

PATHOPHYSIOLOGY

The World Health Organization has identified that the most common cause of female infertility is the failure to ovulate [1,18]. Ovarian quality and quantity steadily decrease as a woman ages and the rate of follicle loss is known to increase in the mid-30s [23]. However, smoking cigarettes is the most significant external factor associated with decreased follicular quantity, ovarian insufficiency, or ovarian resistance owing to hypergonadotropic hypoestrogenic anovulation [18]. There is no opportunity for fertilization or pregnancy with hypergonadotropic hypoestrogenic anovulation. Smoking cigarettes alters the cervical mucous, affects uterine receptivity (embryo implantation), increases the rate of endometrial diseases, and contributes to early menopause that occurs younger than 40 years of age [1,14]. Moreover, an inverse relationship exists between ovarian function and the frequency and rate of smoking [3]. Further discussion of disordered physiologic processes associated with infertility is outside the scope of this article. More common risk factors of female infertility include disorders of ovulation (25%), endometriosis (15%), pelvic adhesions (12%), tubal blockage (11%), other tubal/uterine abnormalities (11%), hyperprolactinemia (7%), and idiopathic infertility [18,23]. Table1 lists other commonly identified factors that influence fertility other than tobacco use.

Tobacco use disorder is caused by an individual's dependence on nicotine, which is found in tobacco. The main ingredient in cigarettes is tobacco, a cured, dried leaf from the plant *Nicotiana tabacum* or *Nicotaiana rustica*. Nicotine is a chemical found in tobacco leaves, and is an oily, colorless liquid in pure form. Nicotine is a highly addictive compound that stimulates the release of the neurotransmitter dopamine, creating the transient feeling of pleasure and calmness [24]. Although variable among individuals, cigarette smokers become quickly addicted to nicotine [24,25]. With long-term tobacco use, a smoker's brain experiences an upregulation of nicotinic–acetylcholine receptors, which causes the brain to require increasing amounts of nicotine to operate normally and avoid experiencing withdrawal [24,25]. Cigarette smoking is associated with the rapid delivery (10–60 seconds of inhalation) of nicotine to the brain and is often triggered by lifestyle routines and habits that promote the cycle of the nicotine addiction [24]. Symptoms of withdrawal include difficulty concentrating, nervousness, headaches, weight gain owing to increased appetite, decreased heart rate, insomnia, irritability, and depression. Even with brief periods of smoking cessation (ie, several hours or overnight), a smoker may experience nicotine withdrawal symptoms, such as feelings of irritability, strong cravings or urges to smoke, depression or anxiety, cognitive and attention deficits, sleep disturbances, and increased appetite [26,27]. These symptoms peak

Table 1
Female and gender-neutral factors that affect fertility [1]

Factors that affect female infertility	Potential causes/rationale
Ovarian	Alteration in the frequency and duration of the menstrual cycle
Cervical	Stenosis or abnormality of the mucus–sperm
Uterine	Congenital or acquired defects that affects endometrium or myometrium
Tubal	Congenital or acquired abnormalities or damage to the fallopian tube
Peritoneal	Anatomic defects or physiologic dysfunction
Environmental/occupational	Chemicals, pesticides, and medical treatments (eg, lead, radiation, chemotherapy, ethylene oxide, dibromochloropropane) associated with artificial abortion/early miscarriage, ovarian problems, and early menopause
Substance abuse	Harmful effects related to caffeine, tobacco, marijuana, or other drugs
Lifestyle	Advanced age, stress, excessive or competitive exercise, inadequate diet associated with extreme weight loss or gain
Concomitant medical diagnoses	Polycystic ovarian syndrome, hypothyroidism, hyperthyroidism, primary pituitary hyperprolactemia, menopause, idiopathic infertility

in the first few days, but eventually disappear within 1 month. Symptoms of nicotine toxicity, otherwise known as acute nicotine poisoning, include nausea, vomiting, salivation, pallor, abdominal pain, diarrhea, and cold sweat.

PHYSICAL ASSESSMENT
In a primary care setting, a focused physical examination can be used to identify other potential causes for infertility other than tobacco use disorder. The examination should be conducted with a targeted approach to assess routine records of vital signs, including BMI, along with an inspection and palpation of the head and neck (thyroid), breasts, abdomen and pelvis, and extremities (skin).

Body mass index
Women with a BMI of less than 17 kg/m$_2$ with excessive exercise or abnormal eating behaviors can improve fertility potential by up to 87% with weight gain to achieve a normal BMI [28]. Similarly, women with a BMI of greater than 27 kg/m^2 with anovulation can improve fertility potential by at least 50% with a loss of 10% of body weight [29]. However, a specific BMI is not recommended to achieve fertility [18].

Head and neck
Further confirmation of the patient's smoker status can be achieved by inspecting the lips, oral mucosa, and gums for signs of irritation or ulceration related

to chronic tobacco product use. The lips may also be assessed for bluish–black discoloration. Simple inspection of the teeth may reveal brown or black discoloration suggestive of repeated exposure to tobacco smoke. The patient should also be evaluated for the presence of "smoker's face," which has been defined as premature wrinkling of the face and cobblestone wrinkles on the posterior surface of the neck [30]. Chronic smokers are known to produce matrix metalloproteinases in higher quantities than in nonsmokers [30]. Matrix metalloproteinases degrade collagen, which results in the observed loss of skin elasticity. Further, the proteolytic activity of matrix metalloproteinases has been extensively considered as a contributing factor to endometriosis-related infertility and other human reproductive disorders [30].

In addition, the thyroid is assessed for gland enlargement and the presence of nodules with the patient seated or in a standing position. Untreated thyroid conditions (subclinical, hypothyroidism, and hyperthyroidism) can impair fertility by interfering with ovulation [31]. A normal thyroid is usually invisible on inspection and difficult to palpate. Conversely, an enlarged thyroid is visible and palpable. Documentation for an enlarged thyroid should include an assessment of the goiter's shape, mobility, consistency, and tenderness.

Breast

A clinical breast examination is needed to assess for the presence of any abnormal masses or secretions. Galactorrhea is the production of milk outside of pregnancy. The most common cause of galactorrhea is a tumor in the pituitary gland, which can cause infertility in both men and women owing to the high associated levels of serum prolactin [32,33]. The patient should be examined sitting up and leaning forward. Then, the areolae are gently squeezed with a gloved hand to express fluid from the nipple. The presence of galactorrhea can support a potential cause for female infertility other than smoking, but confirmation may require imaging, blood tests, or an analysis of the discharge from the nipple to see if fat droplets are present in the fluid.

Abdomen and pelvis

An abdominal examination is used to assess for the presence of abnormal masses at the hypogastrium level, the lowest of the 3 median regions of the abdomen. A pelvic examination may also reveal an obvious cause for female infertility. Smoking is associated with an increased risk of squamous cell carcinoma of the cervix, but not of adenocarcinoma [34]. In one study, smoking increased the risk of squamous carcinoma by approximately 50% (RR, 1.50; 95% CI, 1.35–1.66), but did not increase the risk of adenocarcinoma (RR, 0.86; 95% CI, 0.70–1.05) [34].

Abnormal vaginal or cervical anatomy may be observed during inspection or a mass that requires further workup may be identified during palpation of the lower abdomen. The gynecologic examination should also consist of an evaluation of the Bartholin glands, abnormalities of the labia minora and majora, and any lesions that could indicate a sexually transmitted infection [1]. A speculum examination is recommended to obtain cultures for sexually transmitted infections, assess for cervical stenosis, and obtain a sample for a Papanicolaou test, as indicated. The American Society for Colposcopy and Cervical Pathology provides screening guidelines for the prevention and early detection of cervical cancer [35]. A bimanual examination confirms normal anatomy of the vagina and uterus and excludes the presence of uterine fibroids, ovarian masses, or pelvic nodes indicative of endometriosis [36].

Extremities
Signs of androgen excess with hirsutism (excess hair growth in women following a male distribution pattern) or hypertrichosis (excessive hair growth over and above the normal for the age, sex, and race of an individual) may be observed by examining the upper and lower extremities. The skin should also be assessed for the presence of acne. Moreover, an examination of the extremities can exclude the presence of digit malformations, which may indicate congenital defects.

DIAGNOSIS OF FEMALE INFERTILITY AND TOBACCO USE DISORDER
Female infertility
Female infertility is a disease of the reproductive system among women 15 to 49 years of age and is defined by the failure to achieve a clinical pregnancy after 12 months of regular, appropriately timed, unprotected sexual intercourse or therapeutic donor insemination while not lactating in women younger than 35 years of age [4,17,20]. However, earlier evaluation and treatment after 6 months in women older than 35 years of age or if an expedited evaluation is justified based on the woman's medical history and physical findings. This established diagnosis of female infertility was developed based on normal pregnancy rates, which stipulates that 85% of women will conceive within 12 months [18,28]. A clinical pregnancy is documented by ultrasound examination or histopathologic examination [28].

Tobacco use disorder
A diagnosis of tobacco use disorder (previously referred to as nicotine addiction in the *Diagnostic and Statistical Manual of Mental Disorders*, fifth edition) can be made when someone meets 2 or more of the following 11 criteria, occurring within a 12-month period [21,37]:

1. Tobacco is often taken in larger amounts or over a longer period than was intended.
2. There is a persistent desire or unsuccessful efforts to cut down or control tobacco use.
3. A great deal of time is spent in activities necessary to obtain or use tobacco.
4. Craving, or a strong desire or urge to use tobacco.
5. Recurrent tobacco use resulting in a failure to fulfill major role obligations at work, school, or home.

6. Continued tobacco use despite having persistent or recurrent social or interpersonal problems caused or exacerbated by the effects of tobacco (eg, arguments with others about tobacco use).
7. Important social, occupational, or recreational activities are given up or decreased because of tobacco use.
8. Recurrent tobacco use in situations in which it is physically hazardous (eg, smoking in bed).
9. Tobacco use is continued despite knowledge of having a persistent or recurrent physical or psychological problem that is likely to have been caused or exacerbated by tobacco.
10. Tolerance, as defined by either of the following:
    a. A need for markedly increased amounts of tobacco to achieve the desired effect.
    b. A markedly diminished effect with continued use of the same amount of tobacco.
11. Withdrawal, as manifested by either of the following:
    a. The characteristic withdrawal syndrome for tobacco (refer to criteria A and B of the criteria set for tobacco withdrawal).
    b. Tobacco (or a closely related substance, such as nicotine) is taken to relieve or avoid withdrawal symptoms.

DIAGNOSTIC TESTING
Female infertility
Primary care providers can successfully manage female infertility caused by tobacco use disorder [25]. In fact, many causes of infertility are associated with general medical conditions that are typically treated in a primary care setting. Specific diagnostic fertility tests may include ovulation and ovarian reserve testing; serum testing of reproductive, thyroid, and pituitary hormones, hysterosalpingography (radiographs with contrast to detect abnormalities in the uterine cavity), along with pelvic and transvaginal ultrasound imaging [38]. However, these tests are not first-line in the presence of modifiable risk factors that require attention and intervention. Evaluation to determine the potential cause of infertility is completed initially with basic testing followed by more advanced testing as indicated.

A basic investigation for female infertility includes the following:

- A menstrual history to assess ovulation,
- A hysterosalpingogram to assess tubal patency by injecting dye into the cervix under fluoroscopic imaging to visualize the uterus and fallopian tubes, and
- Possibly a pelvic and/or transvaginal ultrasound examination to assess for the presence of any fallopian tube disease or uterine irregularity capable of causing infertility, such as leiomyomas, uterine adhesions, or asymptomatic polyps [18,36].

A transvaginal ultrasound examination can only provide presumptive evidence of ovulation and is not confirmatory [36]. Furthermore, it requires serial ultrasound examinations to show follicular development and disappearance.

Most abnormal results require referral for treatment, but the primary care provider can counsel patients on treatment options. Laparoscopy is performed if the hysterosalpingography result is abnormal and there is a possibility of pelvic adhesions or endometriosis. All advanced testing provides additional evidence to further evaluate the magnitude of infertility.

It is important not to order diagnostic testing that has minimal predictive values or recommend treatments that are not evidence based [36]. A referral to an obstetrician/gynecologist or fertility specialist is always recommended when nonmodifiable risk factors are suspected or the cause cannot be determined based on the preliminary assessment. An immediate referral is warranted if any of the following are present: oligomenorrhea or amenorrhea; known or suspected uterine, tubal, or peritoneal disease; and advanced endometriosis. In these instances, a women's health specialist is better equipped to perform tests on ovarian reserve, ovulatory function, and structural abnormalities [17,28]. In women older than 40 years, a more immediate referral to a women's health or fertility specialist for evaluation and treatment are warranted because a woman's chances of infertility increases as the woman ages [2,17].

Tobacco use disorder

There are a number of questionnaires that seek to qualify smoking status (ie, active, daily or nondaily smoker) and quantify frequency of cigarette consumption based on packs per day [39–41]. Gathering these data informs the primary care provider's treatment and management of tobacco use disorder. Determining if the individual is a "light" or "heavy" smoker and calculating lifetime smoking history (pack-years) provides important information related to the smoker's severity of nicotine addiction and their potential for withdrawal side effects [40,41]. A comprehensive smoking assessment also may predict a smoker's readiness to change, motivation to quit, and even concomitant depression or anxiety. The smoking assessment questionnaires presented are all validated by self-report, can be administered in a short period of time, and are valid and reliable [20,42]. Both the Fagerstrom Test for Nicotine Dependence (FTND) and the Heaviness of Smoking Index are predictive of sustained smoking cessation over time [21,39,40,42]. Other smoking-related surveys used to capture the psychosocial and behavioral dimensions of nicotine addiction include the Readiness to Quit Ladder and Patient Health Questionnaire (PHQ) assessments.

Smoking status

Self-reported smoking status was assessed using a 30-day point prevalence for smoking cessation [42]. Participants were asked to verify if they were smoking every day, some days, or not at all. No attempt was made to biochemically verify smoking cessation because the inpatient tobacco treatment intervention was introduced as a standard of care, a clinical service, and not as a research protocol. Biochemical validation of smoking cessation was also not feasible owing to constraints associated with cost and access to participants at follow-up [42].

Lifetime smoking history (pack-years)

Pack-years is a way to measure the number of cigarettes a person has smoked over a long period of time [42]. It is calculated by multiplying the number of packs of cigarettes smoked per day over time (lifetime smoking history) by the number of years the person has smoked (age of smoking initiation). For example, 1 pack-year is equal to smoking 1 pack per day for 1 year, or 2 packs per day for half a year, and so on.

Fagerstrom test for nicotine dependence

The FTND (Box 1) is a 6-item survey used to assess a smoker's physiologic dependence on nicotine [39,43]. The FTND's yes/no items are scored from 0 to 1 and multiple choice items are scored from 0 to 3. The items are then summed to yield a total score of 0 to 10, and a higher total score reveals a more intense physical dependence on nicotine or nicotine addiction. The FTND is used to evaluate the quantity of cigarette consumption, the compulsion to use, and dependence [39,43].

The Heaviness of Smoking Index

The Heaviness of Smoking Index (see Box 1) is a 2-item survey that was derived from the first 2 items of the FTND [40]. The Heaviness of Smoking Index asks "How soon after you wake up do you smoke your first cigarette?" and "How many cigarettes do you smoke per day?" Self-reported time to first cigarette is negatively associated with cigarettes per day and objective nicotine dependence testing via blood or urine [40,41].

The Readiness to Quit ladder

The Readiness to Quit ladder (Box 2) is a short, face-valid psychological measure that is generalizable for use with diverse populations to assess along a 10-point ordinal response scale [44]. Readiness to change is an important construct based on the transtheoretical model that plays an integral role in behavioral regulation in addiction [44]. Readiness to quit describes an individual's desire, motivation, or intention to stop smoking cigarettes. According to the scale, a score of 10 corresponds with the statement, "I have quit smoking and I will never smoke again," and a score of 1 corresponds with the statement, "I enjoy smoking and have decided not to quit smoking for my lifetime." The ladder attempts to provide a socially acceptable way to indicate lower levels of readiness to consider quitting [44]. Readiness or motivation impacts engagement and willingness to accept treatment recommendations that support smoking cessation, which significantly influences treatment outcomes [44].

The Patient Health Questionnaire

The PHQ-4 (Box 3) is a 4-item, self-reported questionnaire answered on a 4-point Likert-type scale that is used to measure symptom burden, as well as functional impairment and disability associated with depression and anxiety

Box 1: The FTND and the heaviness of smoking index [25,36]

Please answer the following questions:

1. How soon after you wake do you smoke your first cigarette?

    3—Within 5 minutes

    2—6 to 30 minutes

    1—31 to 60 minutes

    0—After 60 minutes

2. Do you find it difficult to refrain from smoking in places where it is forbidden?

    1—Yes

    0—No

3. Which cigarette would you hate to give up?

    1—The first one in the morning

    0—All the others

4. How many cigarettes per day do you smoke?

    0—10 or less

    1—11 to 20

    2—21 to 30

    3—31 or more

5. Do you smoke more frequently during the first hours after waking than during the rest of the day?

    1—Yes

    0—No

6. Do you smoke if you are so ill you are in bed most of the day?

    1—Yes

    0—No

Scoring:

   Total score ranges from 0 to 10; 7 to 10 points = highly dependent; 4 to 6 points = moderately dependent; less than 4 points = minimally dependent.

The HIS consists of FTND items 1 and 4, using the some response scales and calculating the total score using the sum of the scores on those 2 items.

[45]. The purpose of the PHQ-4 is to allow for a brief but accurate measurement of the most significant symptoms and signs of depression and anxiety by combining a 2-item subscale measure that assesses depression (derived from the original 9-item PHQ) with a 2-item subscale measure that assesses anxiety (derived from the 7-item Generalized Anxiety Disorder Scale) [45,46]. A score of 3 or more on either subscale is considered to be positive. An elevated PHQ-4 score is an indicator for further inquiry to establish the

Box 2: Readiness to quit ladder: assessment of motivation [40]

Instructions: Below are some thoughts that smokers have about quitting. On the ladder, circle the one number that shows what you think about quitting. Please read each sentence carefully before deciding.

10	I have quit smoking.
9	I have quit smoking, but I still worry about slipping back, so I need to keep working on living smoke free.
8	I still smoke, but I have begun to change, like cutting back on the number of cigarettes I smoke. I am ready to set a quit date.
7	I definitely plan to quit smoking in the next 30 days.
6	I definitely plan to quit smoking in the next 6 months.
5	I often think about quitting smoking, but I have no plans to quit.
4	I sometimes think about quitting smoking, but I have no plans to quit.
3	I rarely think about quitting smoking, and I have no plans to quit.
2	I never think about quitting smoking, and I have no plans to quit.
1	I have decided not to quit smoking for my lifetime. I have no interest in quitting.

presence or absence of a clinical disorder warranting evaluation and treatment [45]. Elevated scores can be positive for a disorder such as but not limited to bipolar I, bipolar II, cyclothymia, dysthymia, generalized anxiety disorder, social anxiety disorder, panic disorder, obsessive compulsive disorder, or personality disorders. It is also important to understand that a negative screening result does not mean disease is not present, but rather that the likelihood of disease is low [45].

MANAGEMENT OF FEMALE INFERTILITY CAUSED BY TOBACCO DEPENDENCE IN PRIMARY CARE

Treatment overview

Although most smokers want to quit, 85% of smokers who try to stop smoking without implementing evidence-based tobacco cessation treatment interventions relapse as quickly as within the first week [39]. Similarly, female smokers referred for evaluation and treatment of infertility have tried to quit smoking 3 times previously, and only 18% of these women have received advice on smoking cessation from their referring primary care providers [47]. When successful, smoking cessation represents an important part of effective treatment for infertility.

Simple approach to treatment

Primary care providers can effectively facilitate smoking cessation and abstinence among infertile, female smokers by implementing a relatively simple

Box 3: PHQ 4-item tool for anxiety and depression (PHQ-4) [42]

Over the last 2 weeks, how often have you been bothered by any of the following problems?

1. Feeling nervous, anxious or on edge?

   0—Not at all

   1—Several days

   2—More than half the days

   3—Nearly every day

2. Not being able to stop or control worrying?

   0—Not at all

   1—Several days

   2—More than half the days

   3—Nearly every day

3. Little interest or pleasure in doing things?

   0—Not at all

   1—Several days

   2—More than half the days

   3—Nearly every day

4. Feeling down, depressed or helpless?

   0—Not at all

   1—Several days

   2—More than half the days

   3—Nearly every day

Scoring:

   Total score ranges from 0 to 12; 9 to 12 points = severe; 6 to 8 points = moderate; 3 to 5 points = mild; 0 to 2 none

   Anxiety subscale = sum of items 1 and 2 (score range: 0–6)

   Depression subscale = sum of items 3 and 4 (score range: 0–6)

   A score of 3 or greater on each subscale is considered a positive screen.

and inexpensive intervention (Table 2). This simple intervention approach to treat tobacco dependence includes the following [4,7,47–54]:

- Brief, individualized counseling about the health risks associated with smoking that provides basic education concerning the effects of smoking on fertility;
- Self-help material or referral to a stop-smoking program; and
- Delivering consistent individualized support, and routinely monitoring progress toward cessation.

The management approach as described is highly effective in achieving smoking cessation among reproductive-aged women [47]. This treatment

Table 2
Clinical practice suggestions for assisting a reproductive aged patient to stop smoking

Clinical practice recommendations	Suggested implementation action steps
Ask infertile women if they are a tobacco user. Assess tobacco status with multiple-choice questions.	Expand vital signs to include tobacco use. along with blood pressure, heart rate, temperante. respiratory rate, weight, and BMI. Which of the following statements best describes your cigarette smoking? I smoke regularly now; about the same as before trying to get pregnant. I smoke regularly now, but I've cut down since trying to get pregnant. I smoke every once in a while. I have quit smoking since trying to get pregnant. I wasn't smoking around the time I started trying to get pregnant, and I don't currently smoke cigarettes.
Give clear, strong advice to quit as soon as possible, and encourage abstinence among those who have quit on their own.	Provide encouragement via social support and educational messages/handouts about the impact of smoking on fertility and reproductive health. Advice should be clear, strong, and personalized: "It is important that you quit smoking now, and I can help you." "Occasional or light smoking is still dangerous." "As your clinician. I need you to know that quitting smoking is the most important thing you can do to protect your health now and in the future. The clinic staff and I will help you." "Continuing to smoke makes your chances of getting pregnant low, and quitting may dramatically improve your fertility status."
Use motivational interviewing counseling methods to encourage quit attempts. Help the patient with a quit plan. Provide practical problem solving and skills training.	Highlight previous success in cutting back or attempting to quit to encourage behavior change. If no previous quit attempts have been made, discuss ability to overcome some other personal challenge. STAR is used to prepare a patient for quitting: Set a quit date within 2 weeks. Tell your support system you are quitting. Request understanding and encouragement.

(continued on next page)

Table 2
(*continued*)

Clinical practice recommendations	Suggested implementation action steps
	Anticipate challenges to the upcoming quit attempt including nicotine withdrawal symptoms.
	Remove tobacco products from your environment. Make your home smoke free.
	Counseling should emphasize the following:
	Abstinence. Not even a single puff after the quit date.
	Past quit experience. Identify what helped and what hurt in previous quit attempts.
	Anticipate triggers or challenges. Discuss challenges and triggers and how the patient will successfully overcome, avoid, or alter encountering them.
	Alcohol. Advise the patient to consider limiting or abstaining from alcohol while quitting because alcohol is associated with relapse.
	Other smokers in the household. Patients should encourage housemates to quit with them or to not smoke in their presence.
	Social support is necessary for success. Free quitline support is available in most states (1–800-QUIT-NOW).
Provide education, self-help material, and/or referral to a stop-smoking program. Discuss the limited use of US Food and Drug Administration–approved medications. Arrange for follow-up assessments of tobacco status, including further encouragement of cessation.	Educational handouts should be obtained from national quitline or federal agencies and be culturally/racially/educationally/age-appropriate for the patient. Go to: http://www.smokefree.gov.
	Follow-up contact should begin soon after the quit date, preferably during the first week. A second follow-up contact is recommended within the first month.
	Relapse rates are high among recent quitters in the absence of at least monthly follow-up anchor evidence-based treatment methods.
	Be prepared to reapply tobacco cessation interventions. Recognize that patients may continue or deny smoking. Further encouragement of cessation will be required.

approach increased the proportion of nonpregnant women who quit smoking from 4% at baseline to 24% after 12 months of intervention when encouragement was given during each regularly scheduled follow-up clinic visit according to the patient's individual stage of readiness to quit [47].

The first step in the intervention is an assessment of the patient's tobacco use status. Primary care providers can easily assess for interest and gain buy-in by asking 2 key questions during an encounter to evaluate cause for infertility: "Do you smoke?" and "Do you want to quit?" However, the use of multiple-choice questions (see Table 2) can improve disclosure by 40% [42]. Also, the severity of nicotine addiction and tobacco dependence can be assessed by asking an additional 2 Heaviness of Smoking Index questions: "How soon after you wake up do you smoke your first cigarette?" and "How many cigarettes do you smoke per day?" [40].

After the assessment of tobacco use status is complete, the provider should initiate individualized counseling intended to encourage the patient to move toward a positive behavior change. Motivational interviewing, a counseling approach that focuses on the ambivalence that a person has in initiating or sustaining changes in health-related behaviors, has been effective in influencing smoking cessation efforts or a significant reduction in the number of cigarettes smoked per day [55]. By using ladder scales like the Readiness to Quit Ladder (see Box 2), readiness or internal motivation to quit smoking can be quantified and provide context for behavior that supports smoking cessation efforts [55]. This brief counseling session should provide education about the health consequences of smoking related to infertility and also emphasizes the evidence that decreased smoking increases the potential for future fertility [3,56]. Providing individualized preconception advice on which lifestyle factors may impact fertility and acknowledgment of the reversible dose-dependent relationship between smoking and infertility can be powerful incentives to quit for infertile women who smoke [57].

The information and advice provided during the treatment intervention should be reinforced with resources that support and assist healthy behavior change toward smoking cessation. For example, use of the PHQ-4 (see Box 3) may uncover signs or symptoms of anxiety and/or depression that can potentially complicate coping strategies necessary to overcome a nicotine addiction. Also, self-help handouts or more in-depth educational materials may be given to patients to review at their own convenience. However, a more effective strategy to ensure that ongoing support is maintained is to establish a referral to a smoking-cessation program like the state-funded quitline (1–800-QUIT-NOW) or federally funded text and email programs (go to smokefree.gov) [7]. Finally, this simple, individualized management approach to treat tobacco dependence and improve female infertility requires routine monitoring for progress every 1 to 2 weeks with either an in-clinic or telephone follow-up [7,47,56].

Tobacco treatment options

For the general public, the US Public Health Service considers varenicline (Chantix), sustained-release bupropion (Wellbutrin), and combination nicotine replacement therapy (NRT; ie, transdermal nicotine patch in combination with nicotine gum, lozenge, inhaler, or spray) to be first-line therapies for smoking cessation [7,53]. Each of these pharmacotherapeutic approaches are approximately twice as effective as placebo in randomized trials [7]. Yet, there are no evidence-based recommendations to support the use of either medication during pregnancy or for women trying to become pregnant owing to a lack of adequate and well-controlled studies [58]. However, NRT may be reasonable to consider when the likelihood of achieving smoking cessation is high and its benefits seem to outweigh the combined risks of smoking and NRT in potentially pregnant women [4]. Moreover, the use of NRT, bupropion, or varenicline have resulted in a 2-fold increase in the proportion of nonpregnant women able to quit smoking when behavioral approaches failed [4,54].

NRT medication safety must be considered in the context of inconclusive evidence that cessation medications boost abstinence rates in pregnant smokers [7]. In a study used to develop the 2008 clinical practice guideline update to Treating Tobacco Use and Dependence, women treated with nicotine patches or other NRT (eg, lozenges, gum, inhalers) had significantly higher quit rates than did women receiving cognitive behavioral therapy alone. Moreover, pregnant women receiving cognitive behavioral therapy plus NRT were significantly more likely to achieve short-term and long-term abstinence (approximately 30% vs 10%) [7,59]. If the infertile woman chooses to pursue a pharmacotherapeutic treatment approach to assist with tobacco dependence, nicotine patches are recommended with the dose adjusted according to the number of cigarettes smoked per day.

Nicotine is known to contribute to adverse effects during pregnancy, such as preterm labor, and injury to the fetus [7]. Therefore, caution is suggested if continuing NRT after confirmation of a clinical pregnancy. In 1 study, a small but significant increase in congenital malformations was identified among a group of mothers using NRT compared with a retrospective cohort of mothers who instead smoked in the first trimester [60]. Conversely, other studies document concerns about possible undetected spontaneous abortions among continuing smokers. Several studies of brief exposure to nicotine patches or nicotine gum have demonstrated less of a hemodynamic effect in pregnant women and their fetus than those seen with cigarette smoking given the fact that nicotine levels that result from daily inhalation of 10 or more cigarettes are higher than those associated with recommended doses of nicotine gum and patches [7,54,61].

SUMMARY: IMPLICATIONS FOR PRACTICE

The causal relationship between tobacco use disorder and female infertility is well-established and widely accepted in the literature [4,62]. The evidence consists of numerous studies with varying designs and outcome measures along with several comprehensive reviews, and all support the conclusion that smoking has an adverse impact on infertility, independent of other factors [4,15,63–67]. Study findings have also identified that a female smoker's ability to achieve a clinical pregnancy returns to a similar rate as to nonsmokers with smoking cessation, even if cessation occurs within 1 year of attempting conception [62]. Despite this evidence, fewer than one-half of referring primary care providers talk to infertile women about the risks of smoking and even less infertile women are aware of these risks [4,47,64].

The available biological, experimental, and epidemiologic data indicate that up to 13% of infertility may be attributable to cigarette smoking [4]. Moreover, female smokers have 30% lower pregnancy rates compared with patients undergoing fertility treatments who do not smoke [4]. Complications associated with cigarette smoking and female fertility that can directly affect reproductive processes include conception delay, ovarian follicular depletion, endometrial thickness, and an ineffective response to infertility treatments or assisted reproduction [4,62]. Fortunately, several studies demonstrate a dose–response relationship with the number of cigarettes smoked and document a consistent and highly significant trend of decreasing fertility with increasing numbers of cigarettes smoked per day. It was estimated that 5 years after stopping contraception, 10.7% of smokers smoking more than 20 cigarettes a day remained infertile but only 5.4% of nonsmokers remained infertile [62]. It was also found that former smokers did not seem to show any evidence of a decrease in fertility relative to nonsmokers after a 12- to 60-month time period after stopping contraception [63].

In view of the evidence presented, reproductive-aged women should decrease their cigarette consumption or stop smoking when they are attempting to become pregnant [63]. Effective implementation of smoking cessation strategies and recommendations published in the 2008 clinical practice guideline update to Treating Tobacco Use and Dependence are key to mitigating the infertility consequences of smoking [7]. It is important for primary care providers who encounter infertile women to use every opportunity to assess smoking status, provide education to increase awareness of the infertility risks associated with smoking cigarettes, and deliver evidence-based treatment methods to assist with smoking cessation [44].

Tobacco dependence is a chronic disease that often requires repeated interventions and multiple attempts to quit. The simple treatment approach for tobacco dependence presented in this document are both clinically effective and highly cost effective. However, clinicians should remain cognizant that a relapse is likely and that it reflects the chronic nature of substance abuse and dependence [7]. Data suggest that women are more likely to seek assistance in their quit attempts than are men, but may face different stressors and barriers to quitting that may be addressed in treatment [65]. However, the impact of female-specific motives of quitting to improve fertility and reproductive health may increase quit attempts and successful smoking cessation. Also, the likelihood of achieving smoking cessation seems to increase with each quit attempt and health care providers who care for infertile women have an opportunity to help them quit smoking at every clinic visit [4].

CLINICS CARE POINTS
- Smokers are more likely than non-smokers to be infertile.
- Fertility improves with smoking cessation.
- Routine health maintenance encountered are ideal to implement evidence-based smoking cessation interventions.
- Evidence is limited regarding the use of smoking cessation medications among females who are pregnant or trying to become pregnant.

Disclosure

The authors have nothing to disclose.

References
[1] Elizabeth E Puscheck M. Infertility: practice essentials, overview, etiology of infertility 2020. Available at: https://emedicine.medscape.com/article/274143-overview. Accessed September 05, 2020.

[2] Chandra A, Copen CE, Stephen EH. Infertility and impaired fecundity in the United States, 1982-2010: data from the National survey of family growth. Hyattsville (MD): U.S. Department of Health and Human Services, Centers for Disease Control and Prevention, National Center for Health Statistics; 2013.

[3] Westhoff C, Murphy P, Heller D. Predictors of ovarian follicle number. Fertil Steril 2000;74(4):624–8.

[4] Smoking and infertility: a committee opinion. American Society for Reproductive Medicine. Fertil Steril 2018;110:611–8.

[5] United States Public Health Service, Office of the Surgeon General. The health consequences of smoking- 50 yeas of progress. Rockville (MD): U.S. Dept. of Health and Human Services, Public Health Service, Office of the Surgeon General; 2014.

[6] Creamer MR, Wang TW, Babb S, et al. Tobacco product use and cessation indicators among adults — United States, 2018. MMWR Morb Mortal Wkly Rep 2019;68(45): 1013–9.

[7] Fiore M. Treating tobacco use and dependence: 2008 update. Rockville (MD): U.S. Dept. of Health and Human Services, Public Health Service; 2008; https://doi.org/10.1016/j.amepre.2008.04.009.

[8] Hull MG, North K, Taylor H, et al. Delayed conception and active and passive smoking. Fertil Steril 2000;74(4):725–33.

[9] Paszkowski T, Clarke R, Hornstein M. Smoking induces oxidative stress inside the Graafian follicle. Hum Reprod 2002;17(4):921–5.

[10] Zenzes MT, Krishnan S, Krishnan B, et al. Cadmium accumulation in follicular fluid of women in in vitro fertilization-embryo transfer is higher in smokers**Supported by a grant of the Medical Research Council of Canada (MA-10428) (R.F.C.) and the Royal Bank of Canada. Fertil Steril 1995;64(3):599–603.

[11] Polotsky AJ, Allshouse AA, Casson PR, et al. Impact of male and female weight, smoking, and intercourse frequency on live birth in women with polycystic ovary syndrome. J Clin Endocrinol Metab 2015;100(6):2405–12.

[12] Klonoff-Cohen H, Natarajan L, Marrs R, et al. Cigarette smoking as a risk factor for ectopic pregnancy. Hum Reprod 2001;16:1389–90.

[13] Rebar RW. What are the risks of the assisted reproductive technologies (ART) and how can they be minimized? Reprod Med Biol 2013;12(4):151–8.

[14] Ersoy GS, Zhou Y, Inan H, et al. Cigarette smoking affects uterine receptivity markers. Reprod Sci 2017;24(7):989–95.

[15] Augood C, Duckitt K, Templeton AA. Smoking and female infertility: a systematic review and meta-analysis. Hum Reprod 1998;13(6):1532–9.

[16] Jamal A, Agaku IT, O'Connor E, et al. Current cigarette smoking in adults–United States, 2005-2013. MMWR Morb Mortal Wkly Rep 2014;63:1108–12.

[17] Infertility workup for the women's health specialist: ACOG Committee Opinion. Obstet Gynecol 2019;133(6):E3777–84.
[18] Walker MH, Tobler KJ. Female Infertility. [Updated 2020 Mar 27]. In: StatPearls [Internet]. Treasure Island (FL): StatPearls Publishing; 2020 Available from: https://www.ncbi.nlm.-nih.gov/books/NBK556033/ Acessed June 21, 2020.
[19] Florescu A, Ferrence R, Einarson T, et al. Methods for quantification of exposure to cigarette smoking and environmental tobacco smoke: focus on developmental toxicology. Ther Drug Monit 2009;31(1):14–30.
[20] World Health Organization [WHO]. Sexual and reproductive health: infertility definitions and terminology. 2016. Available at: https://www.who.int/reproductivehealth/topics/infertility/definitions/en/. Accessed September 05, 2020.
[21] Engelmann J, Karam-Hage M, Rabius V, et al. Nicotine dependence, in Abeloff's clinical oncology (6th edition). Armitage JO, Doroshow JH, Kastan MB, et al, editors. Philadelphia: Elsevier 2020.
[22] U.S. Department of Health and Human Services. Preventing tobacco use among youth and young adults: a report of the surgeon general. Atlanta (GA): U.S. Department of Health and Human Services, Centers for Disease Control and Prevention, National Center for Chronic Disease Prevention and Health Promotion, Office on Smoking and Health; 2012.
[23] Berga SL, Marcus MD, Loucks TL, et al. Recovery of ovarian activity in women with functional hypothalamic amenorrhea who were treated with cognitive behavior therapy. Fertil Steril 2003;80(4):976–81.
[24] Dani JA, Harris RA. Nicotine addiction and comorbidity with alcohol abuse and mental illness. Nat Neurosci 2005;8(11):1465–70.
[25] Sarokhani M, Veisani Y, Mohamadi A, et al. Association between cigarette smoking behavior and infertility in women: a case-control study. Biomed Res Ther 2017;4(10):1705.
[26] National Institute on Drug Abuse. Substance Use in women DrugFacts. 2020. Available at: https://www.drugabuse.gov/publications/drugfacts/substance-use-in-women. Accessed September 05, 2020.
[27] Diagnostic and statistical manual of mental disorders. 5th edition. Arlington (TX): American Psychiatric Publishing; 2013.
[28] Crosignani PG. Overweight and obese anovulatory patients with polycystic ovaries: parallel improvements in anthropometric indices, ovarian physiology and fertility rate induced by diet. Hum Reprod 2003;18(9):1928–32.
[29] Jokar TO, Fourman LT, Lee H, et al. Higher TSH levels within the normal range are associated with unexplained infertility. J Clin Endocrinol Metab 2017;103(2):632–9.
[30] Barišić A, Pavlić SD, Ostojić S, et al. Matrix metalloproteinase and tissue inhibitors of metalloproteinases gene polymorphisms in disorders that influence fertility and pregnancy complications: a systematic review and meta-analysis. Gene 2018;647:48–60.
[31] Huang W, Molitch M. Evaluation and management of galactorrhea. 2012. Available at: https://www.aafp.org/afp/2012/0601/p1073.html. Accessed September 05, 2020.
[32] Leung A, Pacaud D. Diagnosis and management of galactorrhea. 2004. Available at: https://www.aafp.org/afp/2004/0801/p543.html. Accessed September 05, 2020.
[33] Benowitz NL. Nicotine Dependence. Pharmacol Ther 2009;837–47; https://doi.org/10.1016/b978-1-4160-3291-5.50060-3.
[34] Frumovitz M. Invasive cervical cancer: epidemiology, risk factors, clinical manifestations, and diagnosis. UpToDate. 2020. Available at: https://www.uptodate.com/contents/invasive-cervical-cancer-epidemiology-risk-factors-clinical-manifestations-and-diagnosis. Accessed October 24, 2020.
[35] American Society for Colposcopy and Cervical Pathology. Screening guidelines. 2019. Available at: https://asccp.org. Accessed October 24, 2020.
[36] Flyckt R, Falcone T. Infertility: a practical framework. Cleve Clin J Med 2019;86(7):473–82.

[37] Gu. Treatment for tobacco Use and dependence. 2014. Available at: https://addiction.surgeongeneral.gov/. Accessed September 05, 2020.

[38] National Cancer Institute. Tobacco and the clinician: interventions for medical and dental practice: monograph 5 of smoking and tobacco control series [publication no 95–3693]. Bethesda (MD): US Department of Health and Human Services, National Institutes of Health; 2008.

[39] Heatherton TF, Kozlowski LT, Frecker RC, et al. The Fagerstrom test for nicotine dependence: a revision of the Fagerstrom tolerance questionnaire. Addiction 1991;86(9):1119–27.

[40] Borland R, Yong HH, O'connor RJ, et al. The reliability and predictive validity of the Heaviness of Smoking Index and its two components: findings from the International Tobacco Control Four Country study. Nicotine Tob Res 2010;12(Supplement 1); https://doi.org/10.1093/ntr/ntq03.

[41] Muscat JE, Stellman SD, Caraballo RS, et al. Time to first cigarette after waking predicts cotinine levels. Cancer Epidemiol Biomarkers Prev 2009;18(12):3415–20.

[42] Abrams DB, Niaura R, Brown RA, et al. The tobacco treatment handbook: a guide to best practices. New York: Guilford Press; 2003. p. 33, Adapted by the Center for Tobacco Independence.

[43] US Public Health Service. A clinical practice guideline for treating tobacco use and dependence: a US Public Health Service report. Rockville (MD): US Department of Health and Human Services, Public Health Service; 2000.

[44] Biener L, Abrams DB. The Contemplation Ladder: validation of a measure of readiness to consider smoking cessation. Health Psychol 1991;10(5):360–5.

[45] Löwe B, Wahl I, Rose M, et al. A 4-item measure of depression and anxiety: validation and standardization of the Patient Health Questionnaire-4 (PHQ-4) in the general population. J Affect Disord 2010;122(1–2):86–95.

[46] Kroenke K, Spitzer RL, Williams JB, et al. An ultra-brief screening scale for anxiety and depression: the PHQ–4. Psychosomatics 2009;50(6):613–21.

[47] Sharma R, Biedenharn KR, Fedor JM, et al. Lifestyle factors and reproductive health: taking control of your fertility. Reprod Biol Endocrinol 2013;11(1):66.

[48] Hughes EG, Lamont DA, Beecroft ML, et al. Randomized trial of a "stage-of-change" oriented smoking cessation intervention in infertile and pregnant women. Fertil Steril 2000;74(3):498–503.

[49] Windsor, R. (2011). Reducing racial/ethnic disparities in reproductive and perinatal outcomes: The evidence from population-based interventions. A. Handler, J. Kennelly, N. R. Peacock (Authors), Reducing racial/ethnic disparities in reproductive and perinatal outcomes: The evidence from population-based interventions (pp. 239-269). New York, New York: Springer. https://doi.org/10.1007/978-1-4419-1499-6_11.

[50] Lindqvist R, Lendahls L, Tollbom O, et al. Smoking during pregnancy: comparison of self-reports and cotinine levels in 496 women. Acta Obstet Gynecol Scand 2002;81(3):240–4.

[51] Homan G, Litt J, Norman RJ. The FAST study: Fertility ASsessment and advice Targeting lifestyle choices and behaviours: a pilot study. Hum Reprod 2012;27(8):2396–404.

[52] Curtis KM, Savitz DA, Arbuckle TE. Effects of cigarette smoking, caffeine consumption, and alcohol intake on fecundability. Am J Epidemiol 1997;146(1):32–41.

[53] Pollak KI, Oncken CA, Lipkus IM, et al. Nicotine replacement and behavioral therapy for smoking cessation in pregnancy. Am J Prev Med 2007;33(4):297–305.

[54] Morales-Suárez-Varela MM, Bille C, Christensen K, et al. Smoking habits, nicotine use, and congenital malformations. Obstet Gynecol 2006;107(1):51–7.

[55] National Center for Chronic Disease Prevention and Health Promotion (US) Office on Smoking and Health. The health consequences of smoking—50 Years of progress: a report of the surgeon general. Atlanta (GA): Centers for Disease Control and Prevention (US); 2014. p. 14, Current Status of Tobacco Control. Available at: https://www.ncbi.nlm.nih.gov/books/NBK294306/.

[56] Fredricsson B, Gilwam H. Smoking and reproduction: short and long term effects and benefits of smoking cessation. Acta Obstet Gynecol Scand 1992;71(8):580–92.

[57] Holland AC. Smoking is a women's health issue across the life cycle. Nurs Womens Health 2015;19(2):189–93.

[58] Oncken CA, Kranzler HR. Pharmacotherapies to enhance smoking cessation during pregnancy. Drug Alcohol Rev 2003;22(2):191–202.

[59] Wallach EE, Hughes EG, Brennan BG. Does cigarette smoking impair natural or assisted fecundity?. Health Protection Branch of Health and Welfare Canada, Ottawa, Ontario, Canada. Fertil Steril 1996;66(5):679–89.

[60] Wallach EE, Stillman RJ, Rosenberg MJ, et al. Smoking and reproduction. Fertil Steril 1986;46(4):545–66.

[61] Weisberg E. Smoking and reproductive health. Clin Reprod Fertil 1985;3(3):175–86.

[62] Wesselink AK, Hatch EE, Rothman KJ, et al. Prospective study of cigarette smoking and fecundability. Hum Reprod 2018;34(3):558–67.

[63] Collins GG, Rossi BV. The impact of lifestyle modifications, diet, and vitamin supplementation on natural fertility. Fertil Res Pract 2015;1(11); https://doi.org/10.1186/s40738-015-0003-4.

[64] Howe G, Westhoff C, Vessey M, et al. Effects of age, cigarette smoking, and other factors on fertility: findings in a large prospective study. 1985. Available at: https://www.ncbi.nlm.nih.gov/pmc/articles/PMC1416131/. Accessed September 05, 2020.

[65] Heger A, Sator M, Walch K, et al. Smoking decreases endometrial thickness in IVF/ICSI Patients. Geburtshilfe Frauenheilkd 2018;78(01):78–82.

[66] AWHONN position statement: smoking and women's health. J Obstet Gynecol Neonatal Nurs 2010;39(5):611–3.

[67] Zhu S, Melcer T, Sun J, et al. Smoking cessation with and without assistance. Am J Prev Med 2000;18(4):305–11.

Opioid Use Disorder Screening for Women Across the Lifespan

Ginny Moore, DNP, WHNP-BC[a],*,
Lindsey Baksh, DNP, WHNP-BC[b],
Shaunna Parker, MSN, WHNP-BC[c],
Shelza Rivas, DNP, WHNP-BC, AGPCNP-BC[d]

[a]Vanderbilt University School of Nursing, 461 21st Avenue South, Nashville, TN 37240, USA;
[b]Vanderbilt University School of Nursing, 461 21st Avenue South, 604 Godchaux Hall, Nashville,
TN 37240, USA; [c]Vanderbilt University School of Nursing, 461 21st Avenue South, 603A Godchaux Hall, Nashville, TN 37240, USA; [d]Vanderbilt University School of Nursing, 461 21st
Avenue South, 602 Godchaux Hall, Nashville, TN 37240, USA

Keywords

• Opioid use • Screening methods • Women's health

Key points

• Opioid use disorder exists on a spectrum of severity.
• The consequences of opioid use disorder are devastating for women and their families.
• Owing to biological, gender-related and societal factors, women are at higher risk for opioid use disorder.
• Health care providers should be aware of substance use screening recommendations across the lifespan and use appropriate screening methods for adolescent, childbearing, and senior women.

Opioids are a category of morphine-like drugs legally prescribed for moderate to severe pain management. Although highly effective in relieving pain, the addictive nature of opioids has resulted in a worldwide epidemic of misuse. In 2018, an estimated 128 people were lost daily to opioid overdose [1–3]. The Centers for Disease Control and Prevention estimate that the financial burden of health care, lost employment productivity,

*Corresponding author. 2801 West Linden Avenue, Nashville, TN 37212. E-mail address: ginny.moore@vanderbilt.edu

https://doi.org/10.1016/j.yfpn.2021.01.007

and criminal justice system costs related to opioid use at $78.5 billion per year [3]. The emotional toll on affected individuals and their loved ones is incalculable.

Opioid use disorder (OUD) describes use that produces significant clinical symptoms of impairment and distress. The disorder exists on a spectrum of severity ranging from mild to moderate to severe [1–3]. The incidence of OUD is estimated at 16 million worldwide and 3 million in the United States [2]. Of the total opioid prescriptions in the United States, 65% are for women. Women are at increased susceptibility for OUD owing to a myriad of factors, including a greater likelihood of experiencing chronic pain and using prescription opioids for longer periods of time than men [1,4,5]. To stem the increasing number of women with OUD, it is imperative that health care providers first identify women at risk through screening. This article reviews professional recommendations for screening, discusses the incidence and susceptibility of OUD in women across the lifespan, and identifies OUD screening methods appropriate for use in the adolescent, childbearing, and senior populations.

ADOLESCENT POPULATION
Opioid use among adolescents and young adults is considered a critical health crisis in the United States. The World Health Organization defines adolescence as between the ages of 10 and 19 years old [6]. Trends in opioid misuse among adolescents has fluctuated in the past several years owing to sparse and inconsistent data. Most recent data from the National Survey on Drug Use and Health shows that in 2016 about 3.6% of adolescents between the ages of 12 and 17 years have misused opioids over the past year [7]. The same survey also showed that pain medication misuse had decreased from 9.5% in 2004 to 3.4% in 2018 among high school seniors [7]. Despite this downward trend, adolescent females make up more than one-half of those adolescents who misuse opioids as compared with adolescent males [4,7].

Several psychosocial factors contribute to higher rates of opioid misuse among adolescent females. Girls at this age begin to engage in intimate partner relationships with partners their age or older and, as a result, are at risk for intimate partner violence. Psychological and emotional distress as a result of intimate partner violence often triggers opioid misuse among girls as a means to cope [4]. Adverse childhood experiences are also major contributors to opioid misuse. Housing instability, neglect, substance use disorder among family members, mental illness, domestic violence, and separation of parents are major events for both girls and boys that further increase their risk for opioid use [4]. For adolescent females, childhood and adolescent sexual and physical trauma has a direct correlation with substance misuse. These events followed by post-traumatic stress disorder are far more common in girls and childbearing women who misuse opioids than in boys and older men [4].

Youth who are at increased risk for opioid misuse include adolescents who identify as lesbian, gay, bisexual, and transgender. About 24.3% of high school lesbian, gay, and bisexual adolescents have misused opioids, which is nearly double the rate of heterosexual adolescents at 12.9% [8]. Transgender adolescent girls and young women seem to have similar prevalence of opioid use compared with the US general population prevalence of 12.5% [9]. At-risk youth further include those of various ethnic backgrounds. A recent study found that Black and Hispanic adolescents have a higher prevalence of opioid misuse than White adolescents [10]. Previous data had shown that White adolescents had historically higher prevalence, however, the study suggests a demographic shift as a result of impactful educational efforts among White adolescents [10].

Death by drug overdose is the most serious consequence of opioid misuse and continues to increase among adolescents [2]. Adolescent girls are far more likely than boys between the ages of 12 and 17 to use opioids for nonmedical reasons and are more likely to become dependent on them [4]. Obtaining opioids has become harder for this particular age group. However, they largely obtain opioids from friends or relatives and are less likely to obtain them from by a medical professional [4]. When asked for reasons to seek opioids, most adolescents conveyed increasing stress, anxiety, and physical pain, as well feeling peer pressure to use as main reasons [4].

The American Academy of Pediatrics highlights the unique role that health care providers have in screening for opioid use among adolescents. About 83% of adolescents have contact with a health care provider at least once annually and these visits serve as prime opportunities to screen, discuss, and intervene with adolescents who consume both alcohol and illicit drugs [8]. Screening, Brief Intervention, and Referral is the main concept that health care providers should use as a tool and strategy for screening [11].

The Care, Relax, Alone, Forget, Friends, Trouble tool is a commonly used 6-question screening method that specifically addresses both alcohol and opioid use in adolescents 14 and older [12]. The Brief Screener for Tobacco, Alcohol, and other Drugs asks 3 questions regarding tobacco, alcohol, and marijuana use and, if positive, further questions are asked to gauge use of opioids and other substances among 12- to 17-year-olds [13]. A tool that is similar to Brief Screener for Tobacco, Alcohol and other Drugs is the Screening to Brief Intervention that measures the frequency of tobacco, alcohol, and marijuana use in the same age group [13]. Last, the adolescent version of the Drug Abuse Screening Test is a 20-question tool that identifies adolescents who are misusing psychoactive drugs and yields a score to reflect the degree of the misuse [14].

Opioid misuse among adolescents can lead to major long-term health implications that can persist and worsen in adulthood. Early screening and intervention by health care providers are imperative to prevent adverse health outcomes later in life.

CHILDBEARING POPULATION

Opioid use in women of childbearing age may lead to health consequences for women and their families. Women of childbearing age are between the ages of 15 and 44 years. Substance use, including opioid use, is most prevalent in this age group [15]. Opioid use in women of childbearing age may be the result of prescribed or nonprescribed opioid pain relievers, illicit use, or medications used for addiction treatment. In the United States, nearly one-half of all pregnancies are unplanned. Given this fact, the use of opioids during the childbearing years places women and their offspring at risk for adverse pregnancy outcomes [16–18]. Providers who care for women with reproductive capability should assess for pregnancy status, sexual activity that may result in pregnancy, desire for pregnancy in the next 12 months, and contraceptive use [18].

The use of opioid medications in childbearing women is increasing. Between 2008 and 2012, the Centers for Disease Control and Prevention found that 28% of privately insured women and 39% of Medicaid insured women filled a legal opioid prescription. Approximately 10% of nonpregnant women age 15 to 44 years report currently using illicit substances, and 5% of pregnant women report substance use in the past month [19]. Prescription drug misuse, including opioids peaks in early adulthood (age 18–25), and then begins to decrease as women approach age 40 [20].

The US Preventative Services Task Force recommends screening all adults over the age of 18 for illicit drug use annually. Additionally, the American College of Obstetricians and Gynecologists, Association of Women's Health Obstetric and Neonatal Nurses, and Centers for Disease Control and Prevention recommend universal verbal screening for drug use in all women of childbearing age [17].

The purpose of screening for substance use in women of childbearing age is to identify those who have or are developing a use disorder [18]. Health care providers should use screening tools that have been adapted and tested in women. Hospitals and clinics should develop screening protocols to ensure that all women are asked about substance use before and during pregnancy. Rates of opioid use are similar among White and Black individuals; however, the rates of death from opioid overdose are higher among Black individuals compared with Whites [21]. Despite the opioid epidemic beginning in rural areas, OUD affects urban, rural, and suburban women [15]. Sexual minority women report misusing opioids at higher rates than their heterosexual counterparts and may be more likely to use heroin. Very little is known about transgender people of childbearing age; however, transgender youth and women may also be at increased risk [22]. Providers should avoid screening for substance use based on risk factors because this practice may lead to stereotyping and will result in missed opportunities for intervention [17,23]. All screening encounters should occur in a private, one-on-one setting. To ensure patient autonomy, patients should be informed of any mandatory reporting laws in their state [23].

Screening begins by informing the woman that every patient is asked about substance use [23]. Practice settings have several options when determining which screening tool to use. In nonpregnant women, the Two Item Conjoint Screening Tool and Cut down, Annoyed, Guilty, Eye-opener – Adapted to

Include Drugs have a high sensitivity and specificity, screen jointly for drug and alcohol use, can be self-administered, and are not time intensive. The Two Item Conjoint Screening Tool asks patients if they have ever drunk more alcohol or used more drugs than intended, and if they have ever felt the need to cut down on drinking or drug use [24]. The Cut down, Annoyed, Guilty, Eye-opener – Adapted to Include Drugs screening asks patients 4 questions related to drug and alcohol use. With both of these screening tools, a single yes response should prompt the provider to consider a substance use disorder and to engage in further assessment [25].

Providers who care for pregnant women should identify a screening tool that has been validated in pregnancy. The Care, Relax, Alone, Forget, Friends, Trouble screening tool for adolescents and young adults (15–24) described in the previous section has been validated in pregnant women of the same age [20]. The American College of Obstetricians and Gynecologists recommends the 5P's and the National Institute of Drug Abuse Quick Screen [15]. The 5P's is a commonly used tool because it was developed for use during pregnancy and screens for both alcohol and drug use. The 5P's asks the woman 5 questions related to use of alcohol or drugs (Parents, Partner, Peers, Personal, Pregnancy), may be self-administered, and is time efficient; however, permission must be obtained to use it [18,23]. The National Institute of Drug Abuse Quick Screen asks patients about past year drug use. If the patient answers yes to any substance, the National Institute of Drug Abuse Modified ASSIST (Alcohol, Smoking and Substance Involvement Screening Test), an 8-question tool should be completed to determine the woman's level of risk for a substance use disorder [26]. Additionally, the Tolerance, Worried, Eye-Opener, Amnesia, K-Cut Down, a 5-item tool, and Tolerance – Annoyance, Cut Down, Eye-Opener, a 4-item tool, commonly used in primary care settings, have both been validated for use during pregnancy [23].

All providers who care for women during the childbearing years must engage in strategies to mitigate the consequences of opioid use. Women who are pregnant are more likely to abstain from substance use than nonpregnant women; however, high rates of unplanned pregnancy and delayed identification of pregnancy may result in fetal exposure to opioids and other illicit substances. Health care providers must use evidence-based opioid prescribing guidelines, provide well-woman or preconception care, and engage in universal screening for OUD to identify women who are at risk for or have OUD.

SENIOR POPULATION

The ages vary according to the source when defining seniors or the older adult population. The US Census Bureau defines the senior population as age 65 and over [27–29]. Older adults are at the greatest risk for adverse effects related to substance use owing to the normal aging physiologic changes that take place in their bodies. Previously, older adult women had lower rates of substance use when compared with adolescents and women of childbearing age. The rates of substance use by older adults and the number at risk for its unhealthy use will increase [30]. This change is due to the large Baby Boomer generation (birth years 1946–1964), who have higher reported rates of substance use and changing attitudes toward alcohol and recreational use of illegal drugs [30].

Although alcohol remains one of the most used substances among older adults, opioid use among older adult women continues to increase. Research indicates that in 2018 26.1% of women compared with 23.5% of men aged 65 and over had at least 1 opioid prescription filled [27–29]. Additionally, data findings suggest that patients prescribed opioids within 7 days of hospital discharge are almost 50% more likely to continue receiving opioid prescriptions approximately 1 year after surgery [31]. There is a higher incidence of opioid prescribing among women owing to the way in which women process pain, a higher likelihood of mental health disorders, greater use of health care, or a higher prevalence of chronic health conditions [28]. Owing to a reported increase in chronic pain disorders such as arthritis and fibromyalgia, women aged 65 and older have a higher percentage of long-term use of prescription opioids than women less than 65 years of age [27–29]. Although further study is needed to completely understand the overall impact of chronic opioid use on chronic conditions, it is apparent that the risks are greater. The likelihood of opioid overdose leading to higher mortality rates among older adult women is increasing. Substance use may have important health impacts, especially among older adults who are at higher risk for chronic diseases and who often take more medications than younger adults [30].

Screening for opioid use occurs less frequently among older adult women when compared with women across the lifespan. OUD often goes unrecognized and untreated in this age group and research on treatment of substance use disorders for this population is limited [32].

There are several factors preventing an accurate assessment of opioid use in the older adult population. As with any age, stigma related to opioid misuse is a major barrier to receiving the appropriate treatment [30]. Both patients and providers may be uncomfortable discussing and reporting stigmatized behavior, such as substance use [30]. Similarly, the clinical manifestations observed with opioid misuse are commonly misinterpreted for the normal aging process. Universal screening is recommended to identify those at risk for or currently engaging in unhealthy substance use behaviors [30].

Data suggest that the recommendations for screening include an approach that is most helpful in identifying opioid use in older adults. The approach for screening focuses on using the appropriate terminology to decrease stigmatizing language that often prevents patients from seeking treatment. According to the data, it is recommended to use the more medically accurate terminology of substance use disorder, unhealthy use, or harmful use and to remove stigmatizing language such as addict, abuser, and addicts [30]. This point is especially important when caring for the older adult population, because historically, individuals in this age group have lived through the punitive language surrounding the war on drugs and may be particularly sensitive to the use of such stigmatizing language, and therefore, not as forthcoming with problems with substance use [30]. Additionally, discussions surrounding alcohol and other substance use should take place in the context of an older adult's overall assessment with the goals of improving health, maintaining function and independence, and improving quality of life [30].

Several screening tools are available that are specific to substance use, including opioid use. However, most of the tools developed are recommended for use with substances, such as alcohol, tobacco, and illicit drugs. Additionally, only a handful of the screening tools were designed specifically for and validated in older adults [30]. The scarcity of screening tools is related to a lack of research pertaining to opioid use in the older adult population. Many of the screening tools have been formatted for screening adolescents and younger adults.

Screening, Brief Intervention, and Referral to Treatment for substance use is a nationwide, evidence-based, public health approach initiative [30]. The Screening, Brief Intervention, and Referral to Treatment strategy has been implemented in a variety of settings, has been adapted for older adults by the Substance Abuse and Mental Health Services Administration, and has the potential to reach the increasing population of older adults who may engage in unhealthy substance use [30]. A screening tool implemented in primary care

Table 1
OUD screening tools

Tool	Length or estimated completion time	Targeted group
5P's (Parents, Partner, Peers, Personal, Pregnancy)	5 questions	Childbearing (pregnant)
Alcohol, Smoking, and Substance Involvement Screening Test (ASSIST)	8 questions	Seniors
Brief Screener for Tobacco, Alcohol and other Drugs	3 questions	Adolescents
Cut down, Annoyed, Guilty, Eye-opener – Adapted to Include Drugs	4 questions	Childbearing (nonpregnant)
CRAFFT (Care, Relax, Alone, Forget, Friends, Trouble)	6 questions	Adolescents and childbearing (pregnant)
Drug Abuse Screening Test	20 questions	Adolescents
NIDA (National Institute of Drug Abuse) Quick Screen	1 question	Childbearing (pregnant)
Screening, Brief Intervention, and Referral to Treatment	5 questions	Seniors
Screening to Brief Intervention	<5 min	Adolescents
Tolerance – Annoyance, Cut Down, Eye-Opener	4 questions	Childbearing (pregnant)
Tolerance, Worried, Eye-Opener, Amnesia, K-Cut Down	5 questions	Childbearing (pregnant)
Two Item Conjoint Screening Tool	2 questions	Childbearing (nonpregnant)

settings, The ASSIST has been used in clinical practice and research but has not yet been validated in older adults [30]. The ASSIST is an interview administered screen with 8 questions that help to assess the level of risk for the previous 3 months and can guide treatment decisions [30].

Opioid use in combination with chronic health conditions predisposes the aging population to a myriad of health risks. There is a lack of supporting evidence related to opioid use in older adults. Because there are screening and treatment limitations surrounding opioid misuse among older adults, further research is necessary.

SUMMARY

OUD is an increasing epidemic with devastating consequences for individuals, their families and communities. Women are at particular risk for OUD owing to biological, gender-related, and societal factors [5]. Early intervention may stem the severity of consequences. Screening of all patients is recommended. A number of tools are available for use in screening. Table 1 summarizes the various tools along with their length and targeted population. Health care providers should be knowledgeable regarding appropriate screening methods for use across the lifespans of the women they serve.

CLINICS CARE POINTS

- The SBIRT method should be used to screen for OUD at every well child visit for adolescents.
- Inform reproductive-age women of state-mandated reporting laws related to prenatal substance use prior to screening for OUD.
- Stigmatizing language should be avoided when providing care to the older adult population.
- Health care providers should talk with older adult patients about opioid use disorder in the same way that other chronic diseases are discussed.

Disclosure

The authors disclose no conflicts of interest.

References

[1] National Women's Health Network. Opioids and women: from prescription to addiction. 2018. Available at: https://www.nwhn.org/prescription-addiction-opioid-epidemic/. Accessed July 25, 2020.
[2] Dydyk AM, Jain NK, Gupta M. Opioid use disorder. Treasure Island (FL): StatPearls Publishing; 2020. Available at: https://www.ncbi.nlm.nih.gov/books/NBK553166/. Accessed July 25, 2020.
[3] National Institute on Drug Abuse. Opioid overdose crisis. 2020. Available at: https://www.drugabuse.gov/drug-topics/opioids/opioid-overdose-crisis. Accessed July 25, 2020.
[4] Office on Women's Health. Final report: opioid use, misuse, and overdose in women. 2017. Available at: https://www.womenshealth.gov/files/documents/final-report-opioid-508.pdf. Accessed July 25, 2020.
[5] National Institute on Drug Abuse. Substance use in women drug facts. 2020. Available at: https://www.drugabuse.gov/publications/drugfacts/substance-use-in-women. Accessed July 25, 2020.

[6] World Health Organization. Recognizing Adolescence. 2014. Available at: https://apps.-who.int/adolescent/second-decade/section2/page1/recognizing-adolescence.html#:~:text=The%20World%20Health%20Organization%20(WHO,the%20age%20of%2018%20years. Accessed July 22, 2020.

[7] U.S. Department of Health and Human Services. Opioids and adolescents 2019. Available at: https://www.hhs.gov/ash/oah/adolescent-development/substance-use/drugs/opioids/index.html. Accessed July 22, 2020.

[8] Youth risk behavior survey – data summary and trends report 2007-2017. Available at: https://www.cdc.gov/healthyyouth/data/yrbs/pdf/trendsreport.pdf. Accessed August 18, 2020.

[9] Restar AJ, Jin H, Ogunbajo A. Prevalence and risk factors of nonmedical prescription opioid use among transgender girls and young women. JAMA Netw Open 2020;3(3):e201015.

[10] Jason AF, Rigg KK. Racial/ethnic differences in factors that place adolescents at risk for prescription opioid misuse. Prev Sci 2015;16(5):633–41.

[11] American Academy of Pediatrics. Committee on substance abuse and prevention. substance use screening, brief intervention, and referral to treatment: policy statement. Pediatrics 2016;138(1):e20161210.

[12] CRAFFT. Get the CRAFFT 2018. Available at: http://crafft.org/get-the-crafft/. Accessed July 22, 2020.

[13] National Institute on Drug Abuse. Screening tools for adolescent substance use 2019. Available at: https://www.drugabuse.gov/nidamed-medical-health-professionals/screening-tools-resources/screening-tools-for-adolescent-substance-use. Accessed July 22, 2020.

[14] European Monitoring Centre for Drugs and Drug Addiction. Drug Abuse Screening Test (DAST-20). 2008. Available at: https://www.emcdda.europa.eu/html.cfm/index3618-EN.html. Accessed July 22, 2020.

[15] Committee on Obstetric Practice. Committee opinion no. 711: opioid use and opioid use disorder in pregnancy. Obstet Gynecol 2017;130(2):e81–94.

[16] Nurse Practitioners for Women's Health. Position statement: prevention and management of opioid misuse and opioid use disorder among women across the lifespan. Washington, DC: HealthCom Media; 2016.

[17] Reddy UM, Davis JM, Ren Z, et al. Opioid Use in Pregnancy, Neonatal Abstinence Syndrome, and Childhood Outcomes Workshop Invited Speakers. Opioid use in pregnancy, neonatal abstinence syndrome, and childhood outcomes: executive summary of a joint workshop by the Eunice Kennedy Shriver National Institute of Child Health and Human Development, American College of Obstetricians and Gynecologists, American Academy of Pediatrics, Society for Maternal-Fetal Medicine, Centers for Disease Control and Prevention, and the March of Dimes Foundation. Obstet Gynecol 2017;130(1):10–28.

[18] Substance Abuse and Mental Health Services Administration. Substance Abuse treatment: addressing the specific needs of women. Treatment Improvement protocol (TIP) Series, No. 51. HHS Publication No. (SMA) 13-4426. Rockville, MD: Substance Abuse and Mental Health Services Administration; 2013.

[19] Ko JY, D'Angelo DV, Haight SC, et al. Vital signs: prescription opioid pain reliever use during pregnancy - 34 U.S. jurisdictions, 2019. MMWR Morb Mortal Wkly Rep 2020;69(28): 897–903.

[20] Schepis TS, Klare DL, Ford JA, et al. Prescription drug misuse: taking a lifespan perspective. Subst Abuse 2020;14:1178221820909352.

[21] Substance Abuse and Mental Health Services Administration. The opioid crisis and the black/African American population: an urgent Issue. Publication No. PEP20-05-02-001. Office of Behavioral Health Equity. Rockville (MD): Substance Abuse and Mental Health Services Administration; 2020.

[22] Girouard MP, Goldhammer H, Keuroghlian AS. Understanding and treating opioid use disorders in lesbian, gay, bisexual, transgender, and queer populations. Subst Abuse 2019;40(3):335–9.

[23] Goodman DJ, Wolff KB. Screening for substance abuse in women's health: a public health imperative. J Midwifery Womens Health 2013;58(3):278–87.

[24] Brown RL, Leonard T, Saunders LA, et al. A two-item screening test for alcohol and other drug problems. J Fam Pract 1997;44:151–60.

[25] Mulvaney-Day N, Marshall T, Downey Piscopo K, et al. Screening for behavioral health conditions in primary care settings: a systematic review of the literature. J Gen Intern Med 2018;33(3):335–46.

[26] NIDA. Resource guide: screening for drug use in general medical settings. National Institute on Drug Abuse website; 2012. Available at: https://archives.drugabuse.gov/publications/resource-guide-screening-drug-use-in-general-medical-settings. Accessed August 14, 2020.

[27] Hunnicutt JN, Chrysanthopoulou SA, Ulbricht CM, et al. Prevalence of long-term opioid use in long-stay nursing home residents. J Am Geriatr Soc 2017;66(1):48–55.

[28] Schieber LZ, Guy GP, Seth P, et al. Variation in adult outpatient opioid prescription dispensing by age and sex — United States, 2008–2018. MMWR Morb Mortal Wkly Rep 2020;69(11):298–302.

[29] Steinman MA, Komaiko KDR, Fung KZ, et al. Use of opioids and other analgesics by older adults in the United States, 1999–2010. Pain Med 2015;16(2):319–27.

[30] Han BH, Moore AA. Prevention and screening of unhealthy substance use by older adults. Clin Geriatr Med 2018;34(1):117–29.

[31] Clarke H, Soneji N, Ko DT, et al. Rates and risk factors for prolonged opioid use after major surgery: population based cohort study. BMJ 2014;348; https://doi.org/10.1136/bmj.g1251.

[32] Prokopczyk-Grol H. Use and opinions among older American adults: sociodemographic predictors. J Gerontol B Psychol Sci Soc Sci 2019;74(6):1009–19.

Pediatrics

Pediatric Pharmacology Update

Teri Moser Woo, PhD, ARNP, CPNP-PC, CNL[a,b,*]

[a]Saint Martin's University, Lacey, WA, USA; [b]ARNP at Convenience Care by Woodcreek Pediatrics – Mary Bridge Children's, Puyallup, WA, USA

Keywords

- Pediatric pharmacology • Pharmacokinetics • History of drug regulation
- Pediatric

Key points

- Most drug regulation legislation in the United States has been proposed to improve drug safety in children, often after a harm to children. Key milestones in US drug regulation have impacted children, from the formation of the Food and Drug Administration in 1906 to the Best Pharmaceuticals for Children Act in 2002.
- The Pediatric Trials Network supports collaboration among pediatric clinical sites and drug trial infrastructure. Enrollment in clinical trials are coordinated among sites to ensure adequate sample size.
- Knowledge of developmental changes in pharmacokinetics in preterm, neonates, and infants are essential to safely prescribe.
- Drug therapy to treat hepatitis C, systemic lupus erythematosus, severe asthma, and moderate to severe atopic dermatitis has expanded age range to include children.

INTRODUCTION

There are more than 156 million medical office visits by children younger than age 15 years annually in the United States, with 18% of children age 0 to 11 years and 27% of adolescents age 12 to 19 years reporting using prescription medication in the past 30 days [1,2]. Nurse practitioners (NPs) who prescribe for children and adolescents need to be knowledgeable of the pharmacokinetics unique to children and use current prescribing recommendations to safely prescribe to this population. This article reviews pediatric drug regulation, pediatric drug trials, pharmacokinetics unique to children and adolescents, and prescribing challenges unique to children and adolescents. Drugs newly approved in

*Saint Martin's University, Lacey, WA. E-mail address: twoo@stmartin.edu

https://doi.org/10.1016/j.yfpn.2021.02.004
2589-420X/21/© 2021 Elsevier Inc. All rights reserved.

children and adolescents, and drugs currently in trials are briefly discussed to provide up-to-date information for the family NP who cares for children.

HISTORY OF PEDIATRIC DRUG REGULATION

Throughout the past century, most drug regulation legislation in the United States has been proposed to improve drug safety in children, often after a harm to children. The US Food and Drug Administration (FDA) was formed in 1906, then the Pure Food and Drug Act was passed regulating interstate commerce of misbranded or adulterated drugs and food, after children died from ingesting tainted food products and soldiers had died from ingesting adulterated quinine [3]. The Federal Food, Drug, and Cosmetic Act was enacted in 1938 due to continued adulteration of products, including sulfanilamide, which had caused more than 100 deaths in children because of the diethylene glycol used in the elixir [4]. The 1938 act mandated truthful labeling and established the new drug application process that required toxicology testing before drugs being promoted and distributed [4]. Thalidomide, a sleeping pill approved for use in Europe in 1956 and distributed to 1000 physicians in the United States under investigational use in 1961, was found to cause significant congenital anomalies. The births of deformed infants whose mothers had taken thalidomide led to the passage of the Kefauver-Harris Amendment in 1962, which mandated preclinical animal trials before testing drugs in humans [4]. The amendment also established 3 phases of clinical testing: Phase I establishes safety and pharmacokinetics; Phase II establishes initial effectiveness and dose range; and Phase III conducts comparative clinical trials [4]. Although the Kefauver-Harris Amendment increased drug safety, it slowed new drug approvals to 8 or 9 years.

In 1983, the Orphan Drug Act passed, which provides developmental grants, a 50% tax credit, and 7-year patent monopoly to encourage pharmaceutical companies to develop drugs for diseases affecting fewer than 200,000 persons including children [4]. The Child Vaccine Act was passed in 1986 requiring patients/parents be informed regarding the vaccines they are being given [5]. In spite of these regulations, in the 1990s more than 70% of medications used in children contained no labeling information for children, leading to the passage of the FDA Modernization Act in 1997 and the "Pediatric Rule" in 1998 [5]. The FDA Modernization Act included a provision extending patent on a drug for 6 months if the manufacture carries out studies in children. The Pediatric Rule required manufactures to conduct pediatric studies to assess safety and efficacy in children [5]. The FDA Modernization Act was challenged by the drug companies and overturned in 2002, a setback for pediatric drug safety.

In 2002, pediatric advocates worked with Congress to get the Best Pharmaceuticals for Children Act passed, which reinstated pediatric exclusivity and amended generic drug approval when pediatric guidelines are added to the labeling [5]. A provision of the Best Pharmaceuticals for Children Act (BPCA) is to consult with pediatric experts to identify and prioritize drugs and therapeutic drug classes to be studied in children and adolescents [6]. The following year, the Pediatric Research Equity Act was signed into law requiring all applications for new active ingredients, new indications, new dosage forms, new dosing regimens, and new routes of administration must contain a pediatric assessment unless the sponsor has obtained a waiver or deferral of pediatric studies [5]. The BPCA was renewed in 2007 and became permanent in 2012 under the FDA Safety and Innovation Act. Milestones in pediatric drug regulation are summarized in Table 1.

PEDIATRIC TRIALS NETWORK

The BPCA is housed in the National Institutes of Health Eunice Kennedy Shriver National Institute of Child Health and Human Development, and has hosted annual meetings of pediatric experts since 2004 to prioritize drugs needing further study. An outcome of the annual meetings of pediatric experts is the development of the Pediatric Trials Network (pediatrictrials.org) funded by the BPCA to allow collaboration among pediatric drug clinical sites and drug trial infrastructure. The Pediatric Trials Network (PTN) addresses challenges in pediatric drug research, including specialized clinical and pharmacology expertise, and pooling of data from multiple sites to obtain sufficient data to obtain valid results in a safe and ethical manner. Since its inception, the PTN has enrolled more than 7000 children in 38 studies of more than 70 drugs. PTN researchers have published more than 50 studies and have submitted pediatric data on 21 medications to the FDA for labeling changes [7]. PTN studies have included antibiotic safety and dosing in premature infants, a long-term antipsychotic safety trial in pediatric patients, drug dosing in obese children, and the use of lorazepam in children with status epilepticus [7]. The PTN POPS (Pharmacokinetics of Understudied Drugs Administered to Children per Standard of Care) study collects a small sample of blood during routine blood draws to study 70 drugs that are already being used as standard of care [8]. Collecting blood samples from patients prescribed targeted medications as part of standard of care is a creative solution to the challenge of studying drugs in infants and children, providing valuable data to expand our understanding of pharmacokinetics in infants and children.

PHARMACOKINETICS IN CHILDREN

Infants, children, and adolescents exhibit developmental differences in pharmacokinetics, affecting drug absorption, distribution, metabolism, and excretion. Knowledge regarding pediatric pharmacokinetics has expanded via studies supported by the PTN. Increased understanding will avoid previous disasters, such as gray baby syndrome caused by inadequate glucuronidation of chloramphenicol, which led to dangerous drug accumulation, and sulfonamide-induced kernicterus in infants caused by displacement of bilirubin from plasma proteins by sulfonamides.

Absorption

Infants and young children have increased absorption through the skin. Preterm infants have an incomplete skin barrier that can be easily penetrated by

Table 1
Milestone in pediatric drug regulation [5]

Year	Regulation	Major provision(s)
1906	Pure Food and Drug Act	• Established the US Food and Drug Administration (FDA) • Regulated interstate commerce of misbranded or adulterated drugs and food
1938	Food, Drug, and Cosmetic Act	• Mandated truthful labeling • Established the new drug application process
1962	Kefauver-Harris Amendment	• Mandated preclinical animal trials before testing drugs in humans • Established 3 phases of clinical testing
1983	Orphan Drug Act	• Tax credits and 7-year patent monopoly, to encourage manufactures to develop drugs for diseases affecting fewer than 200,000 persons
1986	Child Vaccine Act	• Requires vaccine information be given to patients/parents
1997	FDA Modernization Act in 1997	• The FDA could require in writing that the manufacturer submit data on pediatric patients for drugs that appeared to have a pediatric use • Pharmaceutical companies awarded a 6-mo patent extension if they voluntarily tested the medications for safety in children
1998	Pediatric Rule	• Required manufactures to conduct pediatric studies go assess safety and efficacy in children
2002	Best Pharmaceuticals for Children Act (BPCA)	• Pediatric exclusivity • Amended generic drug approval when pediatric guidelines are added to the labeling • Annual list of drugs and therapeutics to receive priority for study in children
2003	Pediatric Research Equity Act	• All applications for new active ingredients, new indications, new dosage forms, new dosing regimens, and new routes of administration must contain a pediatric assessment
2007	Best Pharmaceuticals for Children Act	• BPCA renewed
2012	FDA Safety and Innovation Act	• BPCA became permanent

topical medications [9]. In addition, because infants and children have a greater body surface area to weight than adults, they absorb a proportionally higher dose of medication via the skin than adults [9]. Topical medications known to be more toxic in infants and children include benzocaine and lidocaine (may cause methemoglobinemia), neomycin over large surface areas (ototoxic and neurotoxic), diphenhydramine (altered mental status), doxepin (somnolence), lindane (neurotoxic), and corticosteroids (adrenal suppression) [9]. Care should be taken when prescribing topical medications to infants and children, with clear instructions regarding the amount of drug to apply to the skin and length of treatment.

Distribution

There are changes in body composition in neonates, infants, children, and adolescents. Newborns have total body water (TBW) of 80%, which drops over the first few months to TBW of 60% at 6 months. During puberty, the ratio of fat to lean muscle shifts toward decreased body fat, a shift of approximately 50% in male individuals between 10 and 20 years. Obese children present challenges for dosing due to altered volume of distribution. The PTN has studied pharmacokinetics of drugs in obese children including pantoprazole and clindamycin to determine if obese children with greater volume of distribution require larger doses of medication [7]. The research has determined that pantoprazole should be dosed by lean body weight to prevent increased systemic exposure of pantoprazole [10,11]. Conversely, clindamycin should be dosed by total body weight [12]. The PTN is currently enrolling obese children and adolescents (body mass index greater than the 95th percentile) into a study of dosing of anti-epileptic drugs [7].

Metabolism

Drug metabolism pathways develop variably over childhood. Over the past 20 years, knowledge has increased regarding developmental variation in Phase I and Phase II enzymes leading to differences in how drugs are metabolized. The collaborative work of the PTN has expanded our knowledge of developmental variations in drug metabolism via the PTN POPS study.

Phase I enzymes

The developmental maturation pattern of the cytochrome P450 (CYP450) enzymes varies in the preterm, neonate, infant, and child. Most CYP enzymes have low activity at birth and mature in the first few months of life to adult levels of enzyme activity (Table 2). Some CYP enzymes exceed adult activity during childhood, returning to adult levels as a child enters puberty at Tanner stage II. Dosing adjustments may be required as infants and children go through developmental changes in CYP450 enzyme activity.

Phase II enzymes

Phase II enzymes metabolize water-soluble medications. Commonly used medications such as acetaminophen, morphine, propofol, and caffeine are metabolized via the Phase II enzymes. There is less information regarding Phase II enzyme activity in infants and children than the Phase I enzymes. Morphine is metabolized by the Phase II enzyme glucuronosyltransferase (UGT) 2B7. UGT 2B7 activity is low in preterm infants and neonates leading to decreased plasma clearance of morphine in these populations (see Table 2).

Table 2
Maturation pattern of selected cytochrome P450 (CYP450) enzymes and implications for practice [13,14]

Enzyme	Maturation pattern	Implications for practice
CYP450 1A2	• Absent in fetus and preterm infants • Reaches adult levels at 4 mo of age • Exceeds adult levels at age 1–2 y • At puberty (Tanner Stage II) decreases to adult levels	• Higher doses of medications may be needed from age 2 y until puberty • Monitor therapeutic drug levels during pubertal changes • Erythromycin, phenobarbital, phenytoin, carbamazepine, clarithromycin
CYP450 2D6	• 0% to 5% active at birth • At 2 mo has 20% activity • Reaches adult activity at 3–5 y of age • Significant genetic variability in CYP2D6 activity	• Many psychotropic drugs use CYP2D6 for metabolism • Codeine and dextromethorphan metabolized by CYP2D6 • Breastfed infants may be affected by maternal intake of drugs metabolized by CYP2D6
CYP450 3A4	• Low activity at birth • Reaches 30% to 40% activity by 1 mo • Reaches adult levels by 6 mo of age • Exceeds adult levels at 1–4 y • At puberty (Tanner Stage II) decreases to adult levels	• Many pediatric medications metabolized by CYP2D6 including carbamazepine, prednisone, oral contraceptives, macrolides, nonsteroidal anti-inflammatory drugs, antihistamines • Dosing adjustment based on age • Monitor therapeutic levels, particularly during puberty
UGT 2B7	• Low activity in preterm infants and neonates • Reaches adult levels of activity between 2 and 6 mo; some children do not reach adult activity until age 3 y	• Morphine is metabolized by UGT 2B7

Excretion

The kidneys are immature at birth, with glomerular filtration rates 30% to 40% of adult values, and do not reach adult levels until 6 to 12 months [13]. Drugs that are renally excreted often require lower dosing or altered dosing intervals in neonates and young infants.

PRESCRIBING CHALLENGES IN CHILDREN AND ADOLESCENTS

Prescribing for children and adolescents requires the NP to incorporate the parent into the decision making and education regarding the medication. Infants and young children are totally dependent on the parent or caregiver to administer the medication, therefore inquiring about family schedules and other caregivers is essential for successful treatment. Some children may need 2 prescriptions if the child is going from home to daycare, or between 2 parent's homes in order for all doses to be delivered. Prescribing medication that only requires 1 or 2 doses per day is easier for working parents than medications requiring 3 or 4 doses a day.

Infants and toddlers

Parents of infants and toddlers may need additional education on how to administer a medication. Demonstrating how to administer oral medications with a syringe into the buccal space will empower parents to administer the medication correctly and prevent the infant from spitting out the medication. Toddlers can resist medication administration, and the NP needs to work with parents to find effective medications that need the fewest doses per day and that are palatable whenever possible. Discourage parents from mixing medications in food or drink to administer medications, because if they refuse to finish the mixture there is no way to know how much medication the child has received.

School age and adolescents

School-age and adolescent patients are old enough for the NP to explain the purpose of the medication and cooperate in administration. Ask the child what formulation they prefer: liquid, chewable tablets, or pills to swallow? Be sure a child or adolescent can swallow pills before prescribing. Some medications can be crushed and mixed with highly viscous fluid (eg, chocolate or cherry syrup). Check with the pharmacist before suggesting this if you are not familiar with whether a medication can be crushed.

Before prescribing to school-age children or adolescents, discuss their daily schedule and whether medication would need to be administered at school. School regulations vary regarding administering medication at school. To simplify the medication regimen, avoid school-hour dosing if possible.

Adolescent patients can administer their own medications but have varying amounts of independence in taking their medication. Some adolescents are excellent at medication self-administration, and others have poor adherence. Forming an alliance with the adolescent and parent regarding taking their medication is critical for successful treatment. NPs must know and comply with the laws in their state regarding treating teenagers without parental permission and follow confidentiality laws. Parents may struggle with letting adolescents self-administer their medications, therefore the NP needs to be skilled at assisting families with the developmental transition from parent-controlled to adolescent-controlled medication administration.

NEW DRUG APPROVALS IN CHILDREN

The FDA approved 59 novel drugs in 2018 and 48 in 2019. Of the 48 novel drugs approved in 2019, 20 (42%) were first-in-class, meaning they are a new class of drugs, and 21 (44%) were approved to treat rare or orphan diseases [15]. A number of the newly approved drugs may be used to treat childhood diseases. Elexacaftor/ivacaftor/tezacaftor (Trikafta) was approved in

October 2019 to treat patients 12 years and older who have at least one F508del mutation in the cystic fibrosis (CF) transmembrane conductance regulator (CFTR) gene. Trikafta assists the F508del-CFTR protein function more effectively, progress toward treating the genetic component of CF. Another targeted gene therapy is golodirsen (Vyondys 53) an injectable medication to treat patients with Duchenne muscular dystrophy who have a confirmed mutation of the dystrophin gene amenable to exon 53 skipping. Golodirsen masks exon 53 in the messenger RNA of the Duchenne muscular dystrophy gene so protein synthesis can skip the 52 exon and the remaining exons are able to make a smaller dystrophin protein. Voxelotor (Oxbryta) received accelerated approval in November 2019 to treat children with sickle cell disease. Voxelotor inhibits deoxygenated sickle hemoglobin polymerization so sickle cells are less likely to bind together and form the sickle shape in children with sickle cell disease [15]. Palforzia is a peanut allergen powder for the mitigation of allergic reactions to peanuts in children age 4 to 17 years of age [16].

Several medications expanded their approved age range to children in 2019 and 2020 (Table 3) [16]. Glecaprevir/pibrentasvir (Mavyret), which treats chronic hepatitis C genotype 1, 2, 3, 4, 5, or 6 infection, expanded its indication to adolescents age 12 years and older who weigh at least 45 kg. Sofosbuvir (Sovaldi), which treats chronic hepatitis C genotype 1 or 4 infection and ledipasvir/sofosbuvir (Harvoni) for chronic hepatitis C genotype 1, 4, 5, or 6 infection, both expanded their age range to include patients age 3 to 11 years. Sofosbuvir/velpatasvir (Epclusa) for the treatment of chronic hepatitis C genotype 1, 2, 3, 4, 5, or 6 infection has expanded age range to include children age 6 years and older and at least 17 kg. Belimumab (Benlysta) intravenous infusion for the treatment of patients with active, antibody systemic lupus erythematosus has expanded its indication to include children aged 5 to 17 years. Mepolizumab (Nucala) subcutaneous (SC) injection has been approved for patients age 6 years or older with severe asthma and with an eosinophilic phenotype as add-on maintenance treatment. Safety and efficacy of dupilumab (Dupixent) SC injection has been established in pediatric patients 12 years and older for moderate to severe atopic dermatitis. Colesevelam HCl (Welchol Chewable Bar) has been approved in boys and postmenarchal girls, 10 to 17 years of age, with heterozygous familial hypercholesterolemia as monotherapy or in combination with a statin after failing an adequate trial of diet therapy to reduce low-density lipoprotein cholesterol levels. Safety and effectiveness has been established for topical treatment of acute pain due to minor strains, sprains, and contusions in adults and pediatric patients 6 years and older with diclofenac epolamine (Flector Topical System).

There are several methylphenidate formulations on the market. The newest formulation, Jornay PM, is an extended-release methylphenidate that is administered before bed (6:30 PM to 9:30 PM) [16]. The initial absorption of methylphenidate is no more than 5% during the first 10 hours after taking, then peaks at 14 hours after administration. The delayed peak is designed to peak in the

Table 3
Expanded age ranges for pediatric medications in 2019 and 2020 [16]

Drug	Indication	Age range expansion
Glecaprevir and pibrentasvir (Mavyret)	Chronic hepatitis C genotype 1, 2, 3, 4, 5, or 6 infection	Adolescents 12 y and older or weighing at least 45 kg (kg)
Sofosbuvir (Solvadi)	Chronic hepatitis C genotype 1 or 4 infection	Expanded age range to patients age 3–11 y
Sofosbuvir/velpatasvir (Epclusa)	Chronic hepatitis C genotype 1, 2, 3, 4, 5, or 6 infection	Expanded age range to include children age 6 y and older and at least 17 kg
Ledipasvir and sofosbuvir (Harvoni)	Chronic hepatitis C genotype 1, 4, 5, or 6 infection	Expanded age range to patients age 3–11 y; and at least 17 kg
Belimumab (Benlysta) intravenous infusion	Treatment of patients with active, antibody systemic lupus erythematosus	Expanded to children aged 5–17 y
Mepolizumab (Nucala) subcutaneous (SC) injection	Add-on maintenance treatment of patients with severe asthma and with an eosinophilic phenotype	Extended age ranged down to aged 6 y and older
Dupilumab (Dupixent) SC injection	Moderate to severe atopic dermatitis	Extended age range to age 12 y and older
Colesevelam HCl (Welchol Chewable Bar)	Heterozygous familial hypercholesterolemia as monotherapy or in combination with a statin after failing an adequate trial of diet therapy	Boys and postmenarchal girls, 10–17 y of age
Diclofenac epolamine (Flector Topical System)	Topical treatment of acute pain due to minor strains, sprains, and contusions	Pediatric patients 6 y and older
Ixekizumab (Taltz)	Moderate to severe plaque psoriasis	Labeling extended to include 6–18 y of age
Duloxetine (Cymbalta)	Fibromyalgia in pediatric patients age 13–17 y	Age expanded to patients 13–17 y of age
Crisaborole (Eucrisa) ointment	Mild to moderate atopic dermatitis	Safety and effectiveness have been established in pediatric patients 3 mo and older

morning, often a challenging time for those with attention-deficit hyperactivity disorder.

ONGOING PEDIATRIC DRUG RESEARCH

The PTN has a number of ongoing drug studies designed to study the formulation, dosing, efficacy, and safety of drugs in infants and children. Table 4 lists the ongoing PTN studies and their current status.

Table 4
Ongoing pediatric trials network studies [7]

Pediatric population	Study name and status	Condition
Children age 2–17 y	Anesthetics and Analgesics in children (ANA) – enrolling 120 children	Study of ketamine and hydromorphone to explore PK and safety
Premature infants	Antibiotic safety (SCAMP) -analysis ongoing	Assess safety, efficacy, and PK of a multidrug antibiotic regimen (clindamycin, ampicillin, metronidazole, and piperacillin-tazobactam) for infants with complicated intra-abdominal infections
Obese children 2 to <18 y	Pharmacokinetics of anti-epileptic drugs in obese children (AED) – enrolling	Study of the PK of the antiseizure medications levetiracetam, valproic acid, topiramate, and oxcarbazepine in obese children
Breastfeeding mothers and infants	Pharmacokinetics and Safety of Commonly Used Drugs in Lactating Women and Breastfed Infants (CUDDLE) – enrolling	Ten off-patent drugs will be studied. Enrolling 50 lactating women per drug who are taking one of the drugs as part of their routine care. Drugs to be studied: • Azithromycin • Clindamycin • Escitalopram • Labetalol • Metformin • Nifedipine • Ondansetron • Oxycodone • Sertraline • Tranexamic acid • Ciprofloxacin • Doxycycline • Levofloxacin • Methylphenidate • Sumatriptan
Children <6 mo with single ventricle congenital heart disease	Digoxin – enrollment has started	Pharmacokinetics and safety of digoxin in infants with single ventricle congenital heart disease (CHD)

(*continued on next page*)

Table 4 (continued)		
Pediatric population	Study name and status	Condition
Premature infants	Furosemide – enrolling 120 children at ~30 sites	Assessing safety and effectiveness of furosemide in preterm infants at risk of bronchopulmonary dysplasia
Children age 3–17 y	Long-term Antipsychotic Pediatric Safety Trial (LAPS) – enrolling	2-y prospective observational study to evaluate long-term weight gain with risperidone (350 children) or aripiprazole (350 children)
Children <21 y of age	Pharmacokinetics of Understudied Drugs Administered to Children per Standard of Care (PTN POPS) – enrolling	PK of understudied drugs that are administered to children regularly by their treating physicians; approximately 3000 children, <21 y of age, are participating in the study for up to 90 d
Premature infants	Sildenafil II – enrolling up to 120 patients	Determine effectiveness, PK, and safety of sildenafil in premature infants
Infants	Timolol – analysis ongoing	Evaluating timolol as treatment for infantile hemangioma

Abbreviation: PK, pharmacokinetics.

STAYING UP TO DATE ON NEW PEDIATRIC DRUG DEVELOPMENTS

Staying informed on new pediatric drug developments is critical to providing safe care to children. A reliable resource for updated information is the FDA New Pediatric Labeling Information Database, developed as part of the BPCA and contains updated pediatric labeling in a searchable format [16]. The PTN Web site contains information on ongoing, complete, and published pharmacology studies in children [7].

SUMMARY

Infants, children, and adolescents deserve safe prescribing by knowledgeable NPs. With the expansion of pediatric drug research and new drug approvals, the pediatric provider is challenged with keeping current on new drug approvals and research to provide optimal care. In addition, collaborating with parents is critical for successful pediatric and adolescent drug therapy.

CLINICS CARE POINTS

- Use care when prescribing renally excreted drugs to infants under 6 months of age. Follow dosing guidelines, including avoiding the use of ibuprofen in infants less than 6 months of age.
- Educate parents regarding how to administer an oral medication via oral syringe to infants and toddlers.

References

[1] Centers for Disease Control and Prevention (CDC). National Ambulatory Medical Care Survey: 2016 National Summary Tables. CDC website. 2019. Available at: https://www.cdc.gov/nchs/data/ahcd/namcs_summary/2016_namcs_web_tables.pdf. Accessed July 3, 2020.

[2] Martin CB, Hales CM, Gu Q, et al. Prescription drug use in the United States, 2015–2016. NCHS Data Brief, no 334. Hyattsville (MD): National Center for Health Statistics; 2019. Available at: https://www.cdc.gov/nchs/products/databriefs/db334.htm. Accessed July 3, 2020.

[3] U.S. Food and Drug Administration. Part 1: the 1096 Food and Drugs Act and its enforcement. FDA website 2019. Available at: https://www.fda.gov/about-fda/fdas-evolving-regulatory-powers/part-i-1906-food-and-drugs-act-and-its-enforcement. Accessed July 3, 2020.

[4] U.S. Food and Drug Administration. The history of drug regulation in the United States. 2009. FDA website. Available at: https://www.fda.gov/media/74577/download. Accessed July 3, 2020.

[5] U.S. Food and Drug Administration. Milestones in U.S. food and drug law history. FDA website. 2018. Available at: https://www.fda.gov/about-fda/fdas-evolving-regulatory-powers/milestones-us-food-and-drug-law-history. Accessed July 3, 2020.

[6] Federal Register. Best Pharmaceuticals for Children Act (PBCA) priority list of needs in pediatric therapeutics. 2019. Available at: https://www.federalregister.gov/documents/2019/04/23/2019-08167/best-pharmaceuticals-for-children-act-bpca-priority-list-of-needs-in-pediatric-therapeutics. Accessed July 3, 2020.

[7] Pediatric Trials Network. Available at: https://pediatrictrials.org/our-impact/ Assessed September 7, 2020.

[8] Pediatric Trials Network. Pharmacokinetics of Understudied Drugs Administered to Children per Standard of Care (PTN POPS). Available at: https://pediatrictrials.org/pharmacokinetics-of-understudied-drugs-administered-to-children-per-standard-of-care-ptn-pops/. Accessed July 15, 2020.

[9] Cices A, Bayers S, Verzì AE, et al. Poisoning through pediatric skin: cases from the literature. Am J Clin Dermatol 2017;18(3):391–403. Available at: https://link.springer.com/article/10.1007/s40257-017-0252-6.

[10] Shakhnovich V, Smith PB, Guptill JT, et al. Obese children require lower doses of pantoprazole than nonobese peers to achieve equal systemic drug exposures. J Pediatr 2018;193:102–8.e1.

[11] Shakhnovich V, Abdel-Rahman S, Friesen CA, et al. Lean body weight dosing avoids excessive systemic exposure to proton pump inhibitors for children with obesity. Pediatr Obes 2019;14(1); https://doi.org/10.1111/ijpo.12459.

[12] Smith MJ, Gonzalez D, Goldman JL, et al. Pharmacokinetics of clindamycin in obese and nonobese children. Antimicrob Agents Chemother 2017;61(4):e02014-16.

[13] Kearns GL, Abdel-Rahman SM, Alander SW, et al. Developmental pharmacology—drug disposition, action, and therapy in infants and children. N Engl J Med 2003;349(12):1157–67.

[14] Hines RN. The ontogeny of drug metabolism enzymes and implications for adverse drug events. Pharmacol Ther 2008;118(2):250–67.

[15] U.S. Food and Drug Administration. New drug therapy approvals 2019: advancing health through innovation. 2020. Available at: https://www.fda.gov/drugs/new-drugs-fda-cders-new-molecular-entities-and-new-therapeutic-biological-products/new-drug-therapy-approvals-2019. Accessed March 14, 2021.

[16] U.S. Food and Drug Administration. New Pediatric Labeling Information Database. 2020. Available at: https://www.accessdata.fda.gov/scripts/sda/sdNavigation.cfm?sd=labelingdatabase. Accessed March 14, 2021.

New and Reemerging Infectious Diseases in Pediatrics

Teresa Whited, DNP, APRN, CPNP-PC

University of Arkansas for Medical Sciences, College of Nursing, 4301 West Markham, Little Rock, AR 72205, USA

Keywords
- Infectious disease • Measles • Mumps • Influenza • COVID-19 • Immunization

Key points
- Outbreaks of infectious diseases previously controlled by vaccinations are occurring, especially in patients who are unimmunized or underimmunized.
- Clinicians need to have a high index of suspicion for disease signs and symptoms to limit outbreaks and promote optimal management of infectious diseases in children.
- Many viral illnesses in children require close monitoring and supportive care, such as hydration, isolation precautions, oxygen therapy, and fever management.
- Most disease processes have guidelines for diagnosis and management available through the Centers for Disease Control and Prevention, American Academy of Pediatrics, and others to help guide clinicians in appropriate care.
- Promotion of vaccination and other health promotion measures is essential to prevent or limit infectious diseases in children.

INTRODUCTION

Childhood is a period of rapid growth and development, including the immune system. Children are exposed to a multitude of infections, with one of the leading causes for emergency room visits being respiratory infections [1]. Most infections are viral and self-limiting. However, some infections can have significant complications, such as meningitis, encephalitis, infertility, pneumonia, respiratory failure, and death. It is essential for health care providers to appropriately diagnose and manage these illnesses to prevent significant outbreaks and complications.

E-mail address: tmwhited@uams.edu

https://doi.org/10.1016/j.yfpn.2021.02.005

Clinicians are constantly challenged to diagnose and manage a multitude of emerging and reemerging infections in childhood. Through vaccination programs, many significant diseases with high complication rates have been reduced by 90% or greater [2]. However, outbreaks of vaccine-preventable diseases still occur throughout the United States. Outbreaks often occur in areas of unvaccinated, undervaccinated, or close-proximity populations [2–4]. In the last 10 years, there has been resurgence of measles and mumps with multistate outbreaks resulting in more than 27,000 infections in the last 10 years [3,4]. This resurgence leads to a diagnostic challenge for clinicians to identify diseases not typically seen in practice. In addition, clinicians are faced with ever-evolving diseases such as influenza and COVID-19 (coronavirus disease 2019). This article provides an overview of the diagnosis, management, and prevention of 4 challenging childhood infectious diseases.

MEASLES
History
The typical history of a patient with measles may include a progressively high fever with emergence of upper respiratory symptoms such as rhinorrhea or conjunctivitis [5]. Other symptoms that can be present, especially in younger children, include poor feedings and diarrhea [5]. Often the patient has a chief complaint of a rash following these symptoms. In addition, the history often reveals a lack of measles, mumps, and rubella (MMR) vaccine or only 1 dose of the vaccine [5]. Social history may include close-knit community, school settings, dorms, daycare, or travel to areas of high measles cases [5,6]. In addition, the history may include known exposure to someone with similar symptoms because this disease is highly contagious.

Assessment
Common clinical findings in patients with measles include coryza, conjunctivitis, high fever, lymphadenopathy followed by Koplik spots in the mouth, and finally a rash that begins on the face. Koplik spots are blue-white spots on an erythematous background found on the buccal mucosa [5,6]. Koplik spots can appear 2 to 4 days before or after the onset of the rash [5]. The most characteristic feature of measles is a discrete maculopapular rash that begins at the hairline with progression down the face, neck, and remainder of the body [5,7]. The rash turns brown with initial blanching of the rash [7]. The rash typically is present for approximately 7 days, with resolution of rash followed by desquamation on highly affected areas [5]. If complications do not occur, the disease process is concluded once the rash is resolved.

Pathophysiology
Measles is a very contagious viral infection caused by paramyxovirus [5]. Humans are the only known vectors for this disease process, which remains infectious on contaminated surfaces for only 2 hours [5]. The virus is transmitted primarily through respiratory droplets to the respiratory endothelium of the nasopharyngeal tract [6]. Once within the respiratory system, the virus

replicates quickly and then spreads to other areas of the body. The average incubation period is 10 to 12 days, with rash appearance usually occurring around day 14 of illness [5]. Many patients have upper respiratory symptoms 5 to 7 days into the disease process and are considered contagious until 3 to 4 days after the rash first appears [5]. Approximately 30% of patients experience 1 or more complications, such as pneumonia, seizures, brain damage, and death [5,6].

Diagnosis

Diagnosis should be made through laboratory findings delineated in diagnostic testing. However, measles should be suspected with isolation of the patient with the prodrome associated with measles [5,7].

Differential diagnosis

Differential diagnoses to consider when suspecting measles are primarily viral infections. Many viral infections in childhood result in rashes, including varicella, roseola, erythema infectiosum, and rubella. The distinguishing features of the maculopapular rash beginning on the face and progressing to the remainder of the body with a prolonged rash period of 7 days, brown character, and blanching help to distinguish measles from other rashes [5,7]. In addition, the Koplik spots in the mouth are considered to be pathognomonic for measles [5].

Diagnostic testing

Diagnosis of measles is made through 1 of 3 diagnostic tests. The first is blood immunoglobulin (Ig) G or IgM antibody testing, which indicates an active or recent infection within the last 4 weeks [5,7]. The second way to detect measles is through viral cultures of the throat, nasopharynx, or urine [5,7]. In addition, rapid detection can occur through the use of polymerase chain reaction (PCR) testing. Specimens for PCR can be obtained through the blood, urine, nasopharynx, or throat swabs [5,7]. PCR testing is the preferred method of testing because of the rapid results provided to the clinician [7]. Any suspected cases of measles require immediate reporting to the state health department, a process that varies by state [7].

Management

Management of measles primarily consists of supportive care. However, 2 new recommendations have been highlighted in recent years. The World Health Organization (WHO) and the American Academy of Pediatrics (AAP) recommend vitamin A supplementation in patients who have severe cases, are at high risk for complications, or those who are vitamin A deficient [2,6,7]. Evidence shows vitamin A deficiency can significantly worsen complications of measles and supplementation can reduce the risk of complications such as visual impairment [2,6,7]. The recommended dosing is 50,000 IU for infants less than 6 months, 100,000 IU for infants 6 to 12 months, and 200,000 IU for older children daily for 2 days and then a third dose can be given at 2 to 4 weeks if there is evidence of vitamin A deficiency [2,6,7]. A second recommendation by the

AAP is to provide an MMR vaccine within 72 hours of initial measles exposure and immunoglobulin within 6 days of exposure for patients who do not show adequate immunity to measles [2,7].

Health promotion

Primary prevention for measles is the MMR vaccine. Before initiation of the MMR vaccine, measles accounted for more than 500,000 cases and more than 500 deaths annually [5]. The MMR vaccination program resulted in a 95% reduction in measles cases [5]. However, there has been a resurgence of outbreaks in recent years caused by low vaccination coverage. The Centers for Disease Control and Prevention (CDC) recommends MMR vaccine be administered in 2 doses with the first dose given at 12 to 15 months and the second at 4 to 6 years of age [8]. When 2 doses of MMR are given appropriately, 99% of children show immunity against measles [5,8].

MUMPS

History

History for mumps may include fever, headaches, poor feedings, myalgias, general malaise, or upper respiratory symptoms [9,10]. The classic presenting chief complaint is swelling of the parotid glands [11]. In addition, the history often includes a lack of MMR vaccine or only 1 dose of the vaccine. Social history may include close-knit community, school settings, dorms, daycare, or travel to areas of mumps outbreaks [9]. In addition, the history may include known exposure to someone with similar symptoms because this disease is highly contagious.

Assessment

The primary finding in mumps is unilateral or bilateral parotiditis that usually begins within 2 days of prodrome symptoms [10]. Parotiditis can last for approximately 10 to 14 days [9,10]. Patients can experience edema over the neck, upper chest, and sternum [10]. Mumps can disseminate to other areas of the body, such as the gastrointestinal and genitourinary systems, kidneys, and nervous system, resulting in inflammation of these areas [11]. Systemic complications are more common in older children [10]. Complications can include pancreatitis, orchitis, oophoritis, mastitis, meningitis, encephalitis, and transient or permanent sensorineural hearing loss [10,11]. Although death has not occurred in recent years, infertility can be caused by the orchitis and oophoritis [10,11].

Pathophysiology

Mumps is caused by Paramyxoviridae, which initially replicate in the respiratory epithelia [10]. Humans are the only known vectors, with transmission through respiratory droplets, saliva, or fomites [10]. The most common age group is 2 to 12 years but it can occur at any age [9,10]. Mumps occurs more frequently in winter and spring months and is easily spread to household contacts or those in close proximity [10]. The incubation period of mumps is 12 to 25 days, with parotiditis often occurring 16 to 18 days after exposure [9]. A few patients, such as those who are vaccinated, remain asymptomatic or have a less severe disease process [11]. Patients with mumps are considered contagious 3 days before and 9 days after the parotiditis presents [9,10].

Diagnosis
Diagnosis should be made through laboratory findings delineated in diagnostic testing. However, mumps should be suspected with isolation of the patient with parotiditis and the prodrome associated with mumps.

Differential diagnosis
Mumps can be a cause of parotiditis or swelling in the jaw/neck region. Other differential diagnoses could include bacterial parotiditis, tooth abscess, and lymphadenitis. Definitive diagnosis of mumps cannot be determined without diagnostic testing.

Diagnostic testing
Diagnosis of mumps is made through 1 of 3 diagnostic tests. The first is serum IgM antibody testing, which indicates an active or recent infection within the last 4 weeks [9,10]. The second way to detect mumps is through viral cultures of buccal mucosa or an oral swab [9]. In addition, rapid detection can occur through the use of reverse transcriptase PCR (RT-PCR) testing [10]. Specimens for RT-PCR can be obtained through saliva, urine, or cerebrospinal fluid [9]. The most accurate sample is obtained from the parotid gland, and it may produce false-negatives if it is obtained more than 3 days after onset of parotiditis [9]. To obtain a sample from the parotid gland, it is recommended to massage the gland for 30 seconds and then swab the parotid duct (Stensen duct) [9,10]. RT-PCR testing is the preferred method of testing for suspected cases because of its ability to provide more information about the virus strains [9]. In most states, mumps is a reportable disease to the health department and should be reported even in suspected cases [10,11].

Management
Management of mumps is primarily symptomatic treatment. Recommendations to relieve pain and swelling of parotiditis are analgesics, warm or cold packs, avoidance of foods requiring chewing, and rest [11]. If meningitis symptoms occur, patients may need to be hospitalized for management [9]. Orchiditis is a common complication and should be managed symptomatically with ice, rest, and elevation [9]. If orchiditis occurs, the patient should be monitored closely for signs and symptoms of testicular torsion [9]. Patients with mumps should be excluded from school or childcare for 5 days after parotiditis presentation [10]. If the patient is hospitalized, droplet precautions should be implemented [10]. If exposures are unvaccinated or undervaccinated, these patients should receive the MMR or be excluded for 26 days after the last patient affected by mumps [11].

Health promotion
Primary prevention for mumps is the MMR vaccine. The CDC recommends MMR vaccine be administered in 2 doses, with the first dose given at 12 to 15 months and the second at 4 to 6 years of age [8]. With 2 doses of MMR given appropriately, 88% of children show immunity against mumps [8,10].

INFLUENZA
History
History can show mild to severe symptoms depending on the patient and any complications. The typical history associated with influenza is a rapid onset of fever, nonproductive cough, sore throat, headache, and myalgias [12,13]. Additional symptoms in children can include nausea, vomiting, diarrhea, poor feedings, eye drainage and redness, rhinitis, and increased irritability with poor sleep [13]. History may also include recent exposure to a patient with influenza, other members of the family who are ill with similar symptoms, and school or daycare attendance [12,13].

Assessment
Influenza's associated findings can be mild to severe and based on complications. Common physical examination findings associated with influenza include mild erythema of pharynx, potentially mild to moderate edema of nasopharyngeal structures, and lymphadenopathy in the lymph nodes of the neck [12]. Influenza A is more likely to cause conjunctivitis, crackles associated with pneumonia, abdominal pain, and sputum production [12–14]. Complications frequently occur, especially in patients who are high risk, such as patients with asthma, chronic obstructive pulmonary disease, heart conditions, immunocompromising conditions, and the very young or very old [12]. Complications can include pneumonia, myocarditis, secondary infections, respiratory failure, Guillain-Barré syndrome, multiorgan failure, and death [12].

Pathophysiology
Although influenza is present throughout the year, it has a seasonal peak pattern from December to March in the United States. Influenza has 3 general types: A, B, and C, with multiple subtypes within each type. Each of these types is undergoing antigenic drifts and shifts, which results in new subtypes of the virus. Transmission of influenza in humans occurs from contact with infected persons, their respiratory droplets, or their fomites. Once transmitted, the influenza virus penetrates the epithelial cells of the respiratory tract and replicates. The incubation period of influenza is 1 to 4 days, and the virus is shed for approximately 5 days in respiratory droplets. Patients are considered contagious until fever free for greater than 24 hours and are to be excluded from school, daycare, or other social activities. Influenza can result in significant complications, including systemic illnesses, because it spreads and replicates in vulnerable populations.

Diagnosis

Definite diagnosis of influenza is through diagnostic testing (delineated later). Influenza should be suspected in any patient with typical influenza symptoms, especially during seasonal peaks. Influenza testing is not required in all patients if they are low risk for complications [12]. The CDC algorithm recommends diagnostic testing only in patients whose therapy might be affected by definitive diagnosis, such as hospitalized patients [14]. A clinician can diagnose influenza clinically and treat empirically without definitive diagnostic testing [15].

Differential diagnosis

Differential diagnoses for influenza are viral upper respiratory infection, ear infection, pharyngitis, gastroenteritis, and pneumonia. The distinguishing features of high fever, myalgias, nonproductive cough, and rapid onset help clinicians to identify patients affected by influenza, especially during peak seasons [12,13,15].

Diagnostic testing

Diagnostic testing for influenza comes in 3 types: nucleic acid amplification, antigen detection, and virus isolation [15]. There are multiple manufacturers with a variety of testing methods. Nucleic acid and virus isolation have the highest sensitivity and specificity for influenza, whereas antigen detection has moderate sensitivity but high specificity [15]. Nucleic acid amplification and antigen detection are rapid tests with testing times varying from 10 minutes to 8 hours, whereas virus isolation requires 1 to 10 days [15]. The specimens for diagnostic testing should be collected through nasopharyngeal swab. Because of the possibility of false-negative results, it is recommended to offer treatment of those with an influenza illness and high risk for complications or severe disease [13,15].

Management

According to the CDC and AAP 2019 to 2020 guidelines, the mainstay of therapy for influenza remains symptomatic treatment of all children [15]. For healthy children who have an uncomplicated course, only symptomatic treatment should be offered, with close monitoring for worsening symptoms. However, treatment with oseltamivir is recommended for children who are at risk for complications within 48 hours of symptom onset [15]. It is also recommended at greater than 48 hours in those with severe, worsening, or complicated influenza. Oseltamivir is most effective within 48 hours of onset of symptoms but still has some beneficial efficacy in severe disease [15]. Oseltamivir is approved by the US Food and Drug Administration for children 2 weeks and older; however, it has been used in newborns and preterm infants when the benefits outweigh the risk [15]. Dosing recommendations are as follows: for infants 2 weeks to 1 year of age, 3 mg/kg/dose divided twice a day; 1 to 12 years of age and less than 15 kg, 30 mg twice a day; 15 to 23 kg, 45 mg twice a day; 23.1 to less than 40 kg, 60 mg twice a day; and 1 year of age to adulthood and more than 40 kg, 75 mg twice a day [16]. It is recommended to not delay therapy for confirmatory diagnostic testing in those who need therapy [15].

Health promotion

The best protection provided for influenza is annual vaccination. Because of changes in the virus types annually, the predominant strain varies from year to year and influenza vaccines are manufactured annually to reflect the most common strains for each year [12]. This process leads to the variable efficacy of 50% to 87% for the influenza vaccine [12]. However, even if the influenza vaccine does not prevent the disease, multiple studies have found it reduces the risk of complications and death from influenza in all age groups [12,15]. Influenza vaccine comes in 2 forms: inactivated influenza vaccine (IIV) and live attenuated influenza vaccine (LAIV) [15]. All children aged 6 months or older may receive IIV, whereas only children who are healthy without chronic health conditions such as asthma should receive LAIV [15]. Dosing recommendations for children 6 months to 8 years of age are 2 doses at least 4 weeks apart for initial dosing of vaccine and then 1 dose annually [15]. If the patient is 9 years of age or older, the patient should receive 1 dose annually even if it is the initial time receiving the vaccine [15].

COVID-19

History

The history in children affected by COVID-19 can include exposure to a person diagnosed with COVID-19, lack of appropriate personal protective equipment (PPE) use and social distancing, travel to areas of high infection rates, travel out of state, and attending activities with large crowds or close-proximity conditions [17,18]. A moderate number of children with COVID-19 have no symptoms or very mild symptoms [19]. The most common symptoms in children are fever and/or dry cough [18,19]. Additional symptoms can be chills, fatigue, myalgias, dyspnea, sore throat, rhinorrhea, congestion, nausea, vomiting, and diarrhea [17–19]. A few children develop severe complications, with infants less than 12 months old or those with comorbidities at greatest risk [19]. Complications can include pneumonia, severe respiratory distress, coagulopathies, multiorgan failure, multisystem inflammatory disease, and (rarely) death [20].

Assessment

Based on the evidence reported, most pediatric patients show upper respiratory infection findings such as erythematous, edematous nasopharynx, rhinorrhea, and lymphadenopathy [21,22]. Chest radiograph and chest computed tomography findings can include ground-glass appearance or patchy consolidations in the lungs [21–23]. Many children have normal laboratory findings, with a few showing lymphocytopenia, increased C-reactive protein level, and increased procalcitonin level [20]. A small subset of patients with complications can have coronary aneurysms, multiorgan failure, and pneumonia findings [20–23].

Pathophysiology

Coronaviruses have been present for years and are enveloped positive-strand RNA viruses [22,23]. COVID-19 emerged late in 2019 in Wuhan, China, and is classified as a severe acute respiratory syndrome virus [23]. Full transmission data are not clear but it is known to transmit through respiratory droplets and contact with surfaces that have not been disinfected [21]. COVID-19 virus has been found in stool, urine, blood, semen, and ocular secretions, but no transmission is known to occur through these routes [21]. Patients are considered infectious 1 to 2 days before symptoms and most infectious within the first 7 days of symptoms [21]. The COVID-19 virus can cause symptoms locally, such a mild cold symptoms, or can result in diffuse infection and inflammatory response across the human body.

Diagnosis
Diagnosis is made via diagnostic testing delineated later but should be suspected in patients with upper respiratory infection symptoms, fever, or other common COVID-19 symptoms, especially in those with known exposure to a patient with COVID-19 [23].

Differential diagnosis
Differential diagnoses for pediatric patients with suspected COVID-19 are viral upper respiratory infection, pharyngitis, gastroenteritis, and pneumonia. Clear determination of COVID-19 cannot be confirmed without diagnostic testing.

Diagnostic testing
RT-PCR testing specific to COVID-19 is the standard for identification of infected children [21,22]. Swabbing of the nasopharynx is more effective than throat swabs [21]. Sensitivity of the test is variable from 30% to 80% based on timing of sampling from 4 days after exposure to 7 days into symptoms [21]. The remainder of laboratory testing should be targeted toward the underlying complications associated with COVID-19 [21–23].

Management
Management of COVID-19 is supportive, including symptoms support and oxygen therapy for hypoxia as needed [21,23]. Multiple medications in adult patients are under investigation for management of COVID-19, including antivirals, antibiotics, immunoglobulins, antiinflammatory agents, anticoagulants, hydrochloroquinolone, and immunomodulatory agents [21]. There are few clinical trials in pediatric patients at this time. Limited guidelines for pediatric patients are being evolved but include the following recommendations: supportive treatment according to the patient's clinical needs should be implemented, such as oxygen and hydration support [24]. Systemic corticosteroids, intravenous immunoglobulin, antivirals, and other medications should only be used in the context of clinical trials [24].

Health promotion
Prevention of COVID-19 is primarily focused on limiting exposure to people infected by COVID-19 [21,22]. These measures include avoiding large crowds, social distancing of 2 m (6 feet) or more, wearing a mask or appropriate PPE, excellent handwashing, and disinfection of surfaces to prevent the spread of the virus [21,22]. Guidelines issued by the CDC help guide families, schools,

businesses, and health care providers on best practices for prevention. However, there remains debate and discussion among experts on the best way to prevent COVID-19 because this is an evolving, new pandemic.

SUMMARY

Children represent a vulnerable population to infectious disease. Widespread vaccines can reduce or eliminate the risk of many diseases. However, with suboptimal vaccination status, many previously rare diseases are reemerging, such as measles and mumps. In addition, new and recurrent diseases, such as influenza and COVID-19, continue to challenge clinicians to provide optimal diagnosis and management for children. It is essential for all clinicians to understand outbreak trends of infectious disease processes, have a high index of suspicion for these disease processes where appropriate, and stay up to date on the latest guidelines to manage children affected by infectious diseases. In addition, clinicians need to continue to educate families, schools, and businesses on infection prevention, vaccinations, and other health promotion measures to limit or stop the spread of infectious diseases in children.

References

[1] McDermott K, Stocks C, Freeman W. Statistical brief #242: overview of pediatric emergency department visits 2015. Rockville (MD): Agency for Healthcare Research and Quality; 2018. p. 1–17. Available at: https://www.hcup-us.ahrq.gov/reports/statbriefs/sb242-Pediatric-ED-Visits-2015.pdf.
[2] Wang M, Ratner A. Clinical guideline highlights for the hospitalist: Diagnosis and management of measles. J Hosp Med 2020;15(1):47–8.
[3] Centers for Disease Control and Prevention. Measles outbreaks and cases. 2020. Available at: https://www.cdc.gov/measles/cases-outbreaks.html. Accessed August 19, 2020.
[4] Centers for Disease Control and Prevention. Mumps outbreaks and cases. 2020. Available at: https://www.cdc.gov/mumps/outbreaks.html.
[5] Centers for Disease Control and Prevention. Chapter 13: Measles. Epidemiology and Prevention of Vaccine-Preventable Diseases: Pink Book. 2015: 209-230. Available at: https://www.cdc.gov/vaccines/pubs/pinkbook/meas.html. Accessed August 19, 2020.
[6] Stinchfield P, Orenstein W. Vitamin A for the management of measles in the United States. Infect Dis Clin Pract 2020;28(4):181–7.
[7] Gans H, Maldanado Y. Measles: clinical manifestations, diagnosis, treatment and prevention. Riverwoods (IL): UptoDate; 2019. Available at: https://www.uptodate.com/contents/measles-clinical-manifestations-diagnosis-treatment-and-prevention.
[8] Centers for Disease Control and Prevention. Immunization schedules. 2020. Available at: https://www.cdc.gov/vaccines/schedules/hcp/imz/child-adolescent.html. Accessed August 19, 2020.
[9] Bockelman C, Frawley T, Long B, et al. Mumps: An emergency medicine-focused update. J Emerg Med 2018;54(2):207–14.
[10] Clemmons N, Hickman C, Lee A, et al. Chapter 9: Mumps. Manual for the Surveillance of Vaccine-Preventable Diseases. 2018: 9.1-9.17. Available at: https://www.cdc.gov/vaccines/pubs/surv-manual/chpt09-mumps.html. Accessed August 19, 2020.
[11] Akioyode O, Rungkitwattanakul D, Emezienna N, et al. The resurgence of mumps. US Pharmacol 2019;44(5):18–21.
[12] Centers for Disease Control and Prevention. Chapter12: influenza. Epidemiology and prevention of vaccine-preventable diseases. Atlanta (GA): Pink Book; 2015. p. 187–208.

[13] Kondrich J, Rosenthal M. Influenza in children. Curr Opinions Pediatr 2017;29(3): 297–302.

[14] Centers for Disease Control and Prevention. Guide for considering influenza testing when influenza viruses are circulating in the community. 2019. https://www.cdc.gov/flu/professionals/diagnosis/consider-influenza-testing.htm. Accessed August 19, 2020.

[15] Committee on Infectious Diseases. Recommendations for prevention and control of influenza in children, 2019-2020. Pediatrics 2019;144:1–26.

[16] Epocrates. Pediatric dosing: oseltamivir. Available at: https://online.epocrates.com/results?query=oseltamivir%20peds%20dosing.

[17] Kim L, Whitaker M, O'Halloran A, et al. Hospitalization rates and characteristics of children age <18 years hospitalized with laboratory-confirmed COVID-19-COVID-NET, 14 states, March 1-July 25, 2020. MMWR Morb Mortal Wkly Rep 2020;69(32):1081–8. Available at: https://www.cdc.gov/mmwr/volumes/69/wr/pdfs/mm6932e3-H.pdf.

[18] Ludvigsson J. Systemic review of COVID-19 in children shows milder cases and a better prognosis than adults. Acta Paediatr 2020;109:1088–95.

[19] She J, Liu L, Liu W. COVID 19 epidemic: Disease characteristics in children. J Med Virol 2020;92:747–54.

[20] Viner R, Whittaker E. Kawasaki-like disease: emerging complications during the COVID-19 pandemic. Lancet 2020;395:1741–3.

[21] Wiersinga W, Rhodes A, Cheng A, et al. Pathophysiology, Transmission, diagnosis, treatment of coronavirus disease 2019 (COVID-19). JAMA 2020;324(8):782–93.

[22] McIntosh K. Coronavirus disease 2019 (COVID-19): epidemiology, virology and prevention. Riverwoods (IL): UptoDate; 2020. Available at: https://www.uptodate.com/contents/coronavirus-disease-2019-covid-19-epidemiology-virology-and-prevention.

[23] Centers for Disease Control and Prevention. Interim Clinical Guidance for management of patients with confirmed coronavirus disease (COVID-19). 2020. Available at: https://www.cdc.gov/coronavirus/2019-ncov/hcp/clinical-guidance-management-patients.html. Accessed August 19, 2020.

[24] Liu E, Smyth R, Luo Z, et al. Rapid advice guidelines for management of children with COVID-19. Ann Translational Med 2020;8(10):617–30.

Pain Management in Pediatrics

Elizabeth A. Pasternak, MS-PREP, BSN, RN[a],
Erinn M. Louttit, MSN, FNP-BC[a],
Jennifer J. Wright, MS, CPNP-PC[a], Madison N. Irwin, PharmD[b],
Jessica L. Spruit, DNP, CPNP-AC[a,c,*]

[a]Pediatric Palliative Care, Michigan Medicine, 1540 East Hospital Drive, SPC 4280, Ann Arbor, MI 48109, USA; [b]Department of Pharmacy, Michigan Medicine, University of Michigan College of Pharmacy, 1111 East Catherine Street, Room 324, Ann Arbor, MI 48109, USA; [c]Wayne State University College of Nursing, Michigan Medicine Pediatric Palliative Care, 5557 Cass Avenue, Room 258, Detroit, MI 48202, USA

Keywords

• Pediatric • Pain • Nonpharmacologic • Pharmacotherapy • Opioids

Key points

• Pain is a personal experience, influenced by a variety of factors and biological, psychological, and social interactions.

• Assessment of pain in pediatric patients can be especially challenging given limitations in their ability to communicate experiences; however, various scales are available to assist the health care provider in this assessment.

• Best practice strategies for pediatric pain management include non-pharmacologic and pharmacologic interventions.

• Knowledge of the mechanism of action for each pharmacotherapeutic option guides the health care provider in selecting appropriate agents for each situation.

• Health care providers prescribing controlled substances should be aware of prescription drug monitoring programs and strategies to support patient education and mitigate risk in such circumstances.

*Corresponding author. Wayne State University College of Nursing, Michigan Medicine Pediatric Palliative Care, 5557 Cass Avenue, Room 258, Detroit, MI 48202, USA E-mail address: Jessica.spruit@wayne.edu

https://doi.org/10.1016/j.yfpn.2021.02.002
2589-420X/21/© 2021 Elsevier Inc. All rights reserved.

INTRODUCTION

Pain is a personal experience and varies widely from person to person, and there have been many well-intentioned attempts at definition by experts to capture the intensity of the experience. Perhaps the culture of medicine has contributed to the challenge, with its focus on objectification and identification, and medical training rooted largely in the biological aspects of diseases and conditions, including pain. This challenge becomes particularly heightened in the care of children, who may or not have adequate, or even any, language skills to assist the health care provider (HCP) in understanding their pain experience. Therefore, it is critical that HCP taking care of pediatric patients are knowledgeable about the available assessment tools, recommendations for treatment and management, and how to evaluate effectiveness of their plan in a confident manner. Table 1 provides definitions of types of pain and interventions for pain relief that will be used throughout this article.

Table 1 Key definitions	
Adjuvant [12]	Medications used in addition to first-line medications to enhance
Agonist [27]	Mimics the action of the signal ligand by binding to and activating
Antagonist [27]	Typically binds to receptor without activating, instead decreasing receptor ability to be activated by another agonist
Behavioral health approaches [12]	Focus on psychological factors of the pain experience, including cognition, emotions, behavior, and social factors
Complementary and integrative health [12]	Addition of interventions, such as acupuncture, massage, mind-body behaviors, natural products, meditation, and manipulation (either osteopathic or chiropractic)
Interventional procedures [12]	Subspecialty of pain medicine, uses minimally invasive interventions to alleviate pain and reduce use of oral medications
Mixed pain [12]	Complex overlap of different known types of pain in any combination acting simultaneously and/or concurrently to cause pain in the same body area. It can be either acute or chronic, and clinical prominence of each mechanism may vary at any given point of time
Nociceptive pain [12]	Pain that arises from actual or threatened damage to nonneural tissues and is due to activation of nociceptors
Neuropathic pain [12]	Pain caused by lesion or disease of somatosensory nervous system
Nociplastic pain [12]	Pain arising from altered nociception despite no clear evidence of actual or threatened damage to tissues causing activation of nociceptors or evidence of lesion or disease of the somatosensory nervous system
Restorative therapies [12]	Movement modalities used within multimodal pain care. May be administered by physical and occupational therapists, physiotherapists, and therapeutic exercise

MODELS FOR RECOGNITION OF PAIN
Biopsychosocial model
In modern times, pain is recognized as a universal experience and a public health problem with political implications [1]. In 2011, the National Academy of Medicine (formerly Institute of Medicine) published *Relieving pain in America: a blueprint for transforming prevention, care, education and research* [2]. This statement highlighted the shortfalls in the assessment and treatment of pain that result from gaps in "policy, treatment, attitudes, education, and research." The report called for a "cultural transformation in the way pain is perceived, judged and treated" [2] and defined pain as having sensory, emotional, cognitive, and behavioral components interconnected with environmental, developmental, sociocultural, and contextual factors [2].

More recently, HCP and researchers in the pain field have advocated that advances in understanding pain require a reevaluation of the definition of pain, which was originally created by the International Association for the Study of Pain (IASP) in 1979 [3]. In 2018, the IASP formed a multinational Presidential Task Force consisting of individuals with expertise in clinical and basic science related to pain with the intent to evaluate the current definition. Efforts resulted in a new 2020 revised definition of pain as follows: "an unpleasant sensory and emotional experience associated with, or resembling that associated with, actual or potential tissue damage" [4]. A paramount change in the new definition, compared with the 1979 version, was inserting terminology that acknowledged an individual's ability to describe their experience of pain and for it to be respected [4]. It can be argued the revised definition may lead HCP to inquire how a patient's pain interferes with their daily activities, quality of life (QOL), relationships, and social interactions. Fortunately, the biopsychosocial approach to understanding pain provides an ideal framework for conceptualizing these individual differences in pain.

The biopsychosocial model of pain encapsulates the broader issues embedded in the interactions among the biological, psychological, and social components unique to each patient [5]. Appreciating that the ensemble of biopsychosocial factors contributes to the experience of pain and its expression varies significantly, pain is described as a mosaic of factors that are unique to both an individual and the time it exists in [6].

Within the biopsychosocial model, a major aim of pain treatment is to understand and treat illness within the patient's subjective sense of suffering [7]. Suffering is the perception of a serious threat or damage to one's personal integrity. People in pain frequently report suffering for a multitude of reasons, including "when they feel out of control, when the pain is overwhelming, when the source of the pain is unknown, when the meaning of the pain is dire, or when the pain is chronic" [8]. Unfortunately, acute pain and chronic pain are widespread issues and can have negative impacts on recovery from illness and injury. In addition, poorly managed pain causes unwarranted suffering, adversely impacts QOL, and presents a significant economic cost to society [9].

Kolcaba comfort model

Easing pain should be an elemental human endeavor, and patients should have access to the best level of pain relief that may safely be provided. To assist HCP in application of the biopsychosocial model and interventions to relieve pain, reference to the Theory of Comfort may be helpful. The Theory of Comfort, developed in the 1990s and expanded over the next decades by Katharine Kolcaba, has the potential to place comfort in the forefront of health care. According to Kolcaba, comfort is the product of holistic nursing and is an immediate desirable outcome of nursing care [10]. Kolcaba appreciates the holistic nature of human beings, in that individuals have mental, spiritual, and emotional lives, which are intimately connected with their physical bodies [11].

With the intention to guide assessment, measurement, and evaluation of patient comfort, Kolcaba developed a taxonomy of the concept of comfort. This taxonomy included 3 types of comfort (relief, ease, and transcendence) and 4 contexts in which patient comfort care could occur: physical, psychospiritual, environmental, and sociocultural [10]. Within the model, nursing is described as the process of assessing the patient's comfort needs, developing and implementing appropriate nursing care plans, and evaluating the patient's comfort needs. Assessment should be objective and include intentional evaluation of comfort needs, design of comfort measures to address those needs, and reassessment of comfort levels following implementation [10]. The Comfort Theory provides a foundational and holistic approach to comfort management, which is a priority for patients in all settings.

ASSESSMENT OF PAIN

In pain management, an essential part of providing comprehensive care is a thorough initial evaluation, including assessment of both the medical and the probable biopsychosocial factors causing or contributing to a pain condition [12]. Children and adolescents that can express themselves may describe discomfort or pain and be able to localize and further characterize the unpleasant sensation when asked. However, assessing pain in children can be especially challenging as a result of limitations in their ability to communicate complaints to caregivers. Infants, children, and adolescents may express pain in the form of variable emotion (from withdrawn to crying or angry/aggressive), facial expressions, elevated vital signs, including respiratory rate, heart rate, and blood pressure, and guarding behaviors during assessments or activities. Developmental considerations must also be considered to ensure an accurate assessment of pain [13]. To aid in this, several scales to measure pain experienced in children have been developed and validated [14–17]. A small sample of such scales is described in Table 2. It is important to note additional scales are available and may be more applicable for certain patient populations or health statuses.

Table 2
Pain assessment scales in pediatrics

Scale	Patient age/developmental status	Description of tool	Additional notes
CRIES (crying, requires increased oxygen, increased vital signs, expression, sleeplessness) [14,15]	Neonatal patients	• Observational tool • Considers physiologic (blood pressure, heart rate, oxygen saturation) and behavioral (cry, expression, sleeplessness) components and scores from 0 to 10	• Useful in measuring acute pain, procedural, and postoperative pain, as well as pain in the intensive care unit
Neonatal Infant Pain Scale (NIPS) [14,15]	Preterm and term infants	• Observational tool • Scores facial expression, crying, movement of extremities, state of arousal, and breathing pattern • Scores from 0 to 7	• Useful in procedural pain in neonates
FLACC (face, legs, activity, crying, consolability) [14,16]	Infants, younger children, and children with developmental delays	• Observational tool • Scores each of the categories described in the tool name from 0 to 2, with a higher score indicating greater perceived pain	• Found to be reliable and sensitive in postoperative or postprocedural pain
Faces Pain Scale–Revised (FPS-R) [14]	Children ages 4–12 y old	• Self-report scale • Six faces are presented to the child with various expressions from 0 (no pain) to 10 (very much pain)	• Well-founded reliability, validity, and feasibility in acute and chronic pain • Identified as a preferred scale in children

(continued on next page)

Table 2
(continued)

Scale	Patient age/developmental status	Description of tool	Additional notes
Visual Analog Scale (VAS) [14]	Children and adolescents	• Self-report scale • Children rate their pain by marking the intensity of their pain on a 10-cm line • The length of the line is measured in centimeters to quantify pain severity	• Well-founded reliability, validity, and feasibility in acute and chronic pain
Numerical Rating Scale [14,17]	Children and adolescents	• Self-report scale • Patient rates pain between 0 (no pain) and 5 or 10 (worst possible pain)	• Well-founded reliability, validity, and feasibility in acute and chronic pain • Useful in most children aged 6 and older to assess acute pain • Strong correlations with VAS and FPS-R

APPROACH TO PEDIATRIC PAIN MANAGEMENT
World Health Organization ladder of pain management
In the mid-1980s, recognizing the need for a global standard, the World Health Organization (WHO) brought together a panel of experts who provided the medical community with the analgesic ladder as a framework for decision making regarding treatment of cancer-related pain [18]. The intention was to create a stepwise, thoughtful approach to use the available interventions and medications, including opioids. Over the ensuing decades, this approach has been revised and applied to the management of pain resulting from a wide variety of diagnoses, including adaptation for use in pediatrics [19]. The adult-based analgesic ladder proposes 3 steps, which include a moderate level for which combination products and/or "weak" opioids may be recommended; the adapted pediatric analgesic ladder proposes only 2 steps recognizing contraindications to these medications in this population (Fig. 1). Principles of pain management with analgesics and prescribing remain constant. To support the application of these principles, knowledge of pharmacy resources can be very helpful.

First, analgesics should be delivered by the appropriate route with preference for enteral medications whenever possible. Enteral medications are often very effective, typically lower in cost, easy to obtain, and usually well tolerated with lower risk profile [20]. Although this is the recommendation, excellent symptom management and matching of the route with the individual circumstance are the goals.

Second, attention to providing analgesia at regular intervals in line with individual needs is ideal. For intermittent or unpredictable pain, scheduling medications as needed may be effective and all that is required. However, for more significant and/or lasting pain, scheduling medication around the clock, along with options for as-needed administration for pain that "breaks through," may be indicated for symptom control. When considering dosing intervals, understanding medication profiles, such as half-life and bioavailability, will help to guide decisions [20].

Identification of the level and type of pain guiding initiation and ongoing management within the framework of the WHO 2-step pediatric analgesic pain ladder is the third principle. At any level of the ladder, the level and type of pain are considered. Assessments and recommendations should encompass both pharmacologic and nonpharmacologic approaches to managing pain. Relief plans should include comfort measures, nonopioid or opioid pain medications as appropriate, and thoughtful use of adjuvant medications and interventions intended to enhance therapy. It is important to recognize the "two-way" nature of the analgesic ladder as the pain experience either resolves or encounters exacerbations. The plan is intended to be adaptable and fluid based on ongoing expert assessment [18].

As is consistent with all of health care, every person is unique, and individual needs and responses will vary. Thus, adaptation of the analgesic plan to the individual child is the fourth recommended principle. Although there are

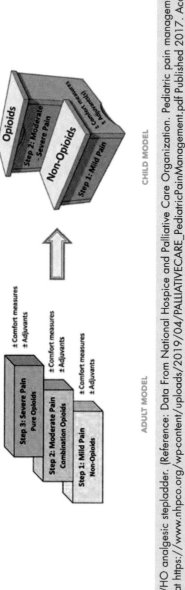

Fig. 1. WHO analgesic stepladder. (Reference: Data From National Hospice and Palliative Care Organization. Pediatric pain management strategies. Available at https://www.nhpco.org/wp-content/uploads/2019/04/PALLIATIVECARE_PediatricPainManagement.pdf Published 2017. Accessed August 11, 2020.)

typically baseline expectations for the level or type of pain that may be experienced in any given situation, the experiences, perceptions, and interpretations of pain are unique to the individual. When caring for children in pain, use of validated assessment tools and clear communication with caregivers most familiar with the child are essential to guide therapy decisions.

Finally, once an appropriate and effective pain management plan is in place, ongoing attention to detail is paramount. Providing thorough education, monitoring, and adaptations as changes occur is essential. It is important to share clear guidelines and parameters for assessment along with expectations for alterations with the child and caregivers. Anticipatory consideration given for next steps in the plan in response to improvements or exacerbations may help to avoid unnecessary delays or crises. The analgesia plan, medications, in particular, should not be extended beyond need nor preemptively discontinued while pain is ongoing [18].

PAIN MANAGEMENT STRATEGIES

Nonpharmacologic interventions

Pain is a multidimensional symptom, and optimal pain management requires a multimodal approach, which should include both pharmacologic and nonpharmacologic therapies. There is pressure for pain medicine to transition from dependence on opioids, ineffective procedures, and surgeries toward comprehensive pain management that includes evidence-based nonpharmacologic options [21]. The current opioid crisis has also triggered intense interest in identifying effective nonpharmacologic approaches to managing pain. In 2019, the US Department of Health and Human Services (HHS) published *Pain management best practices inter-agency task force report: updates, gaps, inconsistencies, and recommendations*, stating HCP are encouraged to consider and prioritize, when clinically indicated, nonpharmacologic approaches to pain management, for improved functionality, activities of daily living, and QOL [12]. For the purpose of this article, restorative therapies, interventional procedures, behavioral health approaches, and complementary and integrative health are discussed as highlighted by the HHS Task Force Report [12].

Restorative therapies

Restorative therapies include treatments provided by physical therapy and occupational therapy professionals, physiotherapy, therapeutic exercise, and other movement modalities. Some examples include massage therapy, cold and heat, traction, and bracing. These interventions can be offered in a variety of settings and can be considered singularly or in combination with other therapies as part of a multimodal approach to the management of acute and chronic pain, depending on the patient. Patient outcomes related to restorative and physical therapies tend to emphasize improvement in outcomes, but there is also value in these therapies helping maintain functionality [12].

Interventional procedures

Interventional pain management is a medical subspecialty that aims to diagnose and treat pain with minimally invasive interventions that can alleviate pain and minimize the use of oral medications [12]. Some examples include (1) peripheral nerve blocks to facilitate physical therapy or relieve neuropathic, musculoskeletal, and sickle cell crisis pain; (2) trigger point injections for myofascial pain syndrome or headache; and (3) intra-articular steroid injections for children and adolescents with juvenile idiopathic arthritis [22,23]. Image-guided interventional procedures (using ultrasound, fluoroscopy, and so forth) can help identify the sources and generators of pain. Diagnostic and therapeutic interventional techniques can be beneficial before extensive surgery, before initiation of opioid therapy, or used in conjunction with other treatment modalities. Although these procedures vary in degree of complexity and invasiveness, many are available on an outpatient basis and have been practiced for decades. There is increasing evidence available to support the utilization of such interventions in the pediatric population [22,23]. A successful outcome depends on whether the intervention is used to treat short-term, acute flares or is part of a long-term management plan, which is patient specific. It is important to note that interventional treatments should be performed by properly trained and certified HCP given associated risks (eg, infection or nerve injury); however, the overall safety and efficacy of such therapies make them an attractive alternative to long-term opioid therapy [12].

Behavioral health approaches

Patient experience and response to pain can be impacted by many psychological factors [12]. Unfortunately, undiagnosed and untreated psychological concerns in patients with pain have negative consequences and are correlated with increased health care utilization and readmissions, decreased treatment adherence, and increased disability. Given the important relationship between pain and psychological health, behavioral health approaches could be considered an essential component of the biopsychosocial model and multidisciplinary pain management, particularly in patient scenarios with chronic pain or concern for acute pain related to somatic conditions. Some examples include (1) cognitive behavioral therapy, (2) mindfulness-based stress reduction, and (3) self-regulatory or psychophysiological approaches, such as biofeedback. Cognitive interventions may include distraction and guided imagery as appropriate for the patient age [24] By addressing the cognitive, emotional, behavioral, and social factors that contribute to pain-related stress and impairment, the goal of behavioral health approaches is to improve the global pain experience and restore function. Treatment should be provided by trained pain psychologists and other HCP that are tailored to address patient preferences and needs [12].

Complementary and integrative health

Complementary and integrative health approaches for pain treatment and management consist of a variety of interventions, but all aim to provide improved relief, when clinically indicated, when used alone or in conjunction with conventional therapies such as medications, behavioral therapies, and interventional treatments. These approaches can include (1) mind-body behavioral interventions, (2) music, (3) acupuncture and massage, (4) osteopathic and chiropractic manipulative therapies, (5) meditative movement therapies, such as yoga and tai chi, and (6) natural products. Ideally, these therapies should be provided or overseen by licensed professionals and trained instructors [12].

The utilization of various therapies depends on the indication, parental interest, and provider knowledge. The American Academy of Pediatrics has published a revised Clinical Report (2017) to guide clinicians caring for children and families who wish to use complementary and integrative therapies [25]. Children and adolescents have successfully engaged in mind-body therapies, such as yoga, to improve symptoms of attention-deficit/hyperactivity disorder, asthma, and juvenile idiopathic arthritis [25]. Therapeutic touch, a biofield therapy, has been successfully applied for reduction of pain and stress in pediatric oncology patients [25]. Massage has been documented across childhood, from the neonatal intensive care unit to infants in an effort to promote weight gain and relieve colic, and to children and adolescents experiencing pain while hospitalized or experiencing depression [25]. Natural products, such as probiotics and fish oil, have been used for infectious/functional diarrhea and neuropsychiatric disorders, respectively [25]. Adolescents use complementary therapies more often than younger children, frequently in the setting of chronic illness, including juvenile idiopathic arthritis, inflammatory bowel syndrome, and mental health conditions [25].

Nonpharmacologic therapies are safe and effective components in comprehensive pain care, and best considered within the context of all evidence-based treatment. They can be stand-alone first line of care interventions or be part of an individualized comprehensive pain care. In addition to being opioid sparing, nonpharmacologic therapies have the "ability to confer additional benefits: a treatment to reduce pain can also reduce anxiety and depression, nausea and vomiting; facilitate restful sleep; and increase a patient's sense of well-being and desire to participate in their own recovery" [21]. Taking this into account, the HCP must be knowledgeable about current pain mechanisms and become familiar with nonpharmacologic modalities and licensed independent practitioners in their system and or area of practice. In addition to recognizing individual health care needs, it is important that the HCP not only assess how a patient manages pain currently and in the past but also reviews which nonpharmacologic strategies they have used and are interested in exploring [21].

PAIN RECEPTORS AND TYPES OF PAIN
Drugs can act as both agonists and antagonists at various receptors, leading both to pain relief and to side effects. Choosing the best medications can be challenging for this reason, especially with interpatient variability in

metabolism and response. Of the medications available to target varying levels and types of pain, few to none are purely active at only 1 receptor. Furthermore, complex processes underlie pain physiology and pathophysiology, making it challenging to achieve total relief of pain without also incurring side effects. These factors complicate development of excellent pain management and symptom control. For example, medications, such as morphine, are very effective in treating significant nociceptive pain resulting from tissue injury; however, morphine acts on multiple receptors. Commonly used pain medications and their receptors are presented in Table 3 [26,27].

OVER-THE-COUNTER PHARMACOTHERAPEUTIC INTERVENTIONS

In treating pediatric patients, the WHO ladder offers evidence-based systematic guidance directing the HCP to start with over-the-counter medications to treat mild pain, such as nonsteroidal anti-inflammatory drugs (NSAIDs) and acetaminophen, both of which have a relatively low side-effect profile at proper doses in younger patients [28]. Again, nonpharmacologic therapies should always be incorporated. In very young children, such as infants, nonpharmacologic methods of pain management are preferred, but acetaminophen can be used. For all children, prescribing principles should aim to use the least effective dose for the shortest period with the presenting problem guiding the practitioner on the anticipated pain timeline. Moderate to severe pain can often be controlled with opioid analgesics. Additional education regarding an appropriate weaning plan is also indicated, as sudden cessation of pain management medications can sometimes lead to a rebound in pain. Clear directions regarding pain signs and symptoms (particularly in young children), doses, frequency, how and when to attempt weaning, and when to call the HCP back are key points to set families up for successfully managing acute pain at home.

Nonsteroidal anti-inflammatory drugs

NSAIDs work by inhibiting cyclooxygenase (COX), an enzyme that transforms arachidonic acid to prostaglandins [29]. There are more than 20 different commercially available NSAIDs classed within 6 groups, and they are roughly divided into 2 categories: short acting (duration of action <6 hours) and long acting (duration of action longer than 6 hours). In addition, they are also often categorized as salicylates, nonselective NSAIDs, and COX-2 inhibitors. At equipotent doses, the NSAIDs have similar efficacy; however, there is notable interpatient variation in response [30]. Although not completely understood, this is likely from the variations in pharmacodynamics, particularly selective potential for COX-1 and COX-2 [31]. NSAIDs have previously not been recommended for use in infants less than 3 months of age because of limited data regarding safety; however, there are new data demonstrating similar safety compared with infants receiving ibuprofen after 3 months of age [32]. Overdose remains the greatest risk of NSAID use in children, and adequate dosing education should be done with special attention paid to concentration [33].

Table 3
Commonly used pain medications and their mechanisms of action

Receptor	Chemical mediator	Medication examples	Mechanism	Common uses
NMDA receptor [26,27]	Glutamate	Ketamine (Ketalar) Methadone (Dolophine)	NMDAR antagonism in the brain and spine	Nociplastic pain
μ-Opioid receptor [27]	Endorphins	Morphine Oxycodone (Oxycontin) Hydromorphone (Dilaudid) Methadone (Dolophine)	μ-Opioid receptor agonism in the brain and spine	Nociceptive pain
α₂ Receptor [26]	Norepinephrine	Dexmedetomidine (Precedex) Clonidine (Catapres)	α₂ receptor agonism in the brain and spine	Neuropathic, nociplastic pain
5-HT receptor [26]	Serotonin	Duloxetine (Cymbalta) Venlafaxine (Effexor) Nortriptyline (Pamelor)	Serotonin and norepinephrine reuptake inhibition in the brain	
α2δ1 subunit of voltage gated Ca²⁺ channels [26]	—	Gabapentin (Neurontin) Pregabalin (Lyrica)	Calcium channel (α2δ1) antagonism in the periphery, brain, and spine	Neuropathic, nociplastic pain
Voltage-gated Na⁺ channels [26]	—	Mexiletine Systemic lidocaine Valproic acid (Divalproex) Topiramate (Topamax)	Sodium channel antagonism in the periphery, brain, and spine	Neuropathic, nociplastic pain
Prostaglandin receptors [26]	Prostaglandins	Ibuprofen (Motrin) Ketorolac (Toradol)	COX-1/2 inhibition prevents synthesis of proinflammatory mediators (prostaglandins)	Nociceptive pain (inflammatory)
Prostaglandin receptors + multiple others [26]	Prostaglandins	Acetaminophen (Tylenol)	Inhibition of prostaglandin synthesis in the brain and spine + other mechanisms that are not well understood	Nociceptive pain (inflammatory)
Prostaglandin receptors [26]	Prostaglandins	Prednisone (Deltasone) Methylprednisolone (Medrol) Dexamethasone (Decadron)	Inhibition of prostaglandin synthesis, reduction of capillary permeability	Nociceptive pain (inflammatory)

Ibuprofen is the most frequently used NSAID in children, with oral-dose guidelines of 4 to 10 mg/kg every 6 to 8 hours not to surpass 40 mg/kg/d. Of note, over the counter labeling advises a maximum dose of 1200 mg/day. Side effects are generally associated with long-term use and include gastrointestinal bleeding and renal toxicity [34]. Long-term use of NSAIDs in children should be done under the supervision of an HCP, and although there is a paucity of data regarding the safety profile of long-term use of NSAIDs in children, 1 large randomized controlled trial demonstrated a similar low rate of adverse events between ibuprofen and acetaminophen when used long term [35]. Aspirin, a salicylate NSAID, is not to be used in febrile or acute illness because of its association with Reye syndrome [36]. The effect on prostaglandins and the subsequent anti-inflammatory properties warrant consideration of NSAIDs for use in pain associated with inflammatory diagnoses, whether as singular therapy or in combination with other pain medications.

Acetaminophen

The mechanism of action of acetaminophen is not well understood, but it is thought to inhibit COX pathways [37]. Although acetaminophen has antipyretic and analgesic properties, it only has weak anti-inflammatory properties [37]. One of the greatest benefits of acetaminophen is that it has a range of ways to be administered: oral, intravenously, or rectal. Oral administration is often used in older children, whereas younger children may benefit from rectal dosing if unable to take oral medications. Oral acetaminophen dose guidelines are 10 to 15 mg/kg every 4 to 6 hours, maximum daily dose or 75 mg/kg/d but not to exceed 4000 mg. Rectal dosing is 10 to 20 mg/kg every 4 to 6 hours, again with maximum daily dose of 75 mg/kg/d and not to exceed 4000 mg [38].

Refractory pain

In the setting of pain that is not relieved by an NSAID or acetaminophen, modification of the pain regimen is necessary. If NSAIDs and acetaminophen have not been trialed before, the first recommendation could be to attempt using both agents as a combination without opioid use for the acute pain episode. It may be presumed that over-the-counter medications are not as strong or beneficial for pain as those available by prescription. However, more recent evidence has shown that nonopioid approaches to pain management can be as effective as opioid medications and have the added benefit of negating serious risks associated with opioid use, including respiratory depression, tolerance, and addiction [39]. In cases whereby this is not a reasonable initial approach to pain control, there is evidence supporting concomitant use of NSAIDs, acetaminophen, and opioids for an opioid-sparing effect [39].

PRESCRIPTION SUBSTANCES

Opioids

Although opiates and opioids are often used interchangeably, there is a notable difference between them. Opiates are drugs naturally derived from opioid poppy plants and include morphine and codeine. Opioids are partially or fully synthetic drugs, with similar mechanisms of action to opiates, and include oxycodone, hydromorphone, fentanyl, and methadone [27]. For the remainder of this article, the term opioid will be inclusive of both opiates and opioids. Opioids work as agonists of the mu, delta, and kappa receptors, with each opioid having individual affinity for those receptors. Side effects commonly associated with opioids, including constipation, euphoria, respiratory depression, and sedation, are also the result of the agonism of these receptors [27]. For moderate to severe pain, short-acting opioids are an appropriate course of treatment with limited supplies of 5 to 7 days. Choosing which opioid to prescribe is based on route preferred for administration, common adverse effects, any prior experiences with opioids, and patient/family preference. Morphine is frequently used in children, as it has the most data and a relatively safe profile [40]. Hydromorphone is more potent than morphine with a quicker onset of action. Some patients report they have less side effects on hydromorphone than with morphine, as morphine is involved with histamine release, which can increase side effects [27]. Oxycodone is also slightly more potent than morphine and has a longer half-life (Table 4).

Opioids to avoid include codeine and tramadol because of a large variability in metabolism in children leading to unpredictable levels of active metabolites and the potential for extreme overdoses [41,42].

CONSIDERATIONS FOR PRESCRIBING
Prescribing principles
With the ongoing opioid epidemic in the United States, there can be heightened trepidation surrounding prescribing and managing opioids. However, using consistent prescribing principles and a systematic way of educating patients and families about their use and the expectations as the HCP, opioids can become a useful tool for primary care providers.

Table 4
Pharmacologic properties of opioids

Medication	Onset of action, min	Peak effect	Half-life, h	Duration, h	Oral dose, mg/kg	Frequency, h
Hydromorphone	15–30	30–60 min	2–3	3–4	0.03–0.06	3–4
Morphine	30	Approx. 1 h	2–6 (longer half-life the younger the child)	3–5	0.3	3–4
Oxycodone	10–15	30 min to 1 h	3–4	3–6	0.1–0.2	4–6

Lexicomp. 2020. Hudson, OH: Lexicomp.

The goal of any pain medication management is to use the lowest dose to achieve acceptable pain control while avoiding unwanted side effects. Therefore, the initial dose is going to depend on the type of pain as determined by the presenting problem, the severity of the pain, and the patient's prior tolerance or intolerance of medications. For acute pain, short-acting oral opioids are typically prescribed every 4 hours, based on their duration of action (see Table 4). As-needed dosing is preferred over scheduled and adjuvants. Acetaminophen and NSAIDs should be considered for use, and they can help decrease opioid use [39]. If unsure how a particular patient will react to a new opioid, it is acceptable to start the prescription at the lower end of the recommended dose and advise the family to be in contact between 24 and 48 hours of use regarding efficacy. Titration may be needed, although unlikely with short courses of therapy. Finally, when starting a new opioid prescription for any patient, discuss opioid-induced constipation and ways to mitigate the development of this uncomfortable side effect. It may be beneficial to recommend a bowel regimen, like senna, be started and continued during the time of opioid use [43].

Important education to cover includes that medications should not be shared, should preferably be kept in a lockbox out of sight, and only the dose prescribed, at the interval prescribed, should be given [44]. In addition, education regarding proper disposal of unused or expired medications should be covered. By visiting www.rxdrugdropbox.org, families can find if their local community hosts a safe drop-off location. If not, advising them to mix the medication with an unpalatable substance like kitty litter or coffee grounds and disposing in the household garbage is acceptable. It is recommended that medications are not crushed at the time of disposal. Remind families to remove all identifying information from the bottle, including patient and medication name [44].

Education for health care providers

In the pediatric age group, the origin of pain conditions is crucial because the developing nervous system can be especially vulnerable to pain sensitization and development of neuroplasticity. Data support that poorly managed pain in children can put them at risk for persistent pain and increased impairment as they transition into adulthood, which could even be linked to the development of new chronic pain conditions [45,46]. Therefore, as the mandate for improved pain management has grown, there is an equal need for better education and training of HCP as well as more time and resources to respond to the unmet needs of patients with painful conditions. Fortunately, there are multiple entities, including academic institutions, health systems, government agencies, nonprofit organizations, and pharmaceuticals manufacturers, that have developed and disseminated pain- and opioid-related patient education programs, toolkits, pamphlets, and other interventions to help deliver effective, patient-centered pain care while reducing the risk associated with prescription opioids [13].

Primary care providers are on the front line of pain—seeing patients every day who are dealing with acute, chronic, or even intractable pain. As a result, it is imperative these HCP establish treatment goals with all patients, including realistic goals for pain and function. Before initiating opioid therapy, HCP should discuss with patients known risks and benefits. HCP may be required to review state prescription drug monitoring program (PDMP) data [44]. PDMPs vary from state to state, but this electronic database of controlled substances dispensed (typically schedule II to IV drugs) is 1 promising tool that can help improve patient safety. These programs allow HCP and pharmacists (and in some states, insurers, researchers, and medical licensing boards) access to the data, monitor use by patients, monitor prescribing practices by HCP, and check population-level drug use trends [13].

HCP can also calculate the total amount of opioids prescribed per day in morphine milligram equivalents (MME) or morphine equivalent daily dosing (MEDD), which helps determine patients who may be at risk for opioid-related complications, especially with potential to overdose. In addition, HCP can view if patients are being prescribed other substances that may increase risk of concomitant opioid use, such as benzodiazepines [47].

For HCP managing chronic pain, the Centers for Disease Control and Prevention (CDC) *Guidelines for prescribing opioids for chronic pain* is a useful tool to guide patient education and prescribing practices [48]. The CDC also has available materials that can be accessed by patients, which may support conversation with HCP when discussing treatment options with all of the risks and benefits carefully being considered. To learn more, please visit: https://www.cdc.gov/drugoverdose/prescribing/guideline.html. Opioid therapy should only continue if meaningful improvement in both pain and function outweighs risk to patient safety [48]. It is important for HCP to assess and provide education surrounding factors that increase risk for opioid overdose, such as history of overdose or substance use disorder, higher opioid dosages ($\geq$50 MME or MEDD per day), or concurrent benzodiazepine use [48].

Identifying patients at risk of substance use disorder will help minimize potential adverse consequences and facilitate treatment or referral if warranted [12]. HCP should also incorporate strategies to mitigate risk into the management plan, which includes offering naloxone. Naloxone, an opioid antagonist, is a medication designed to counteract the life-threatening effects of an opioid overdose. There are currently 3 Food and Drug Administration–approved formulations of naloxone: (1) injectable (*professional training required*); (2) autoinjectable (EVZIO, *a prefilled autoinjection device that makes it easy to inject naloxone quickly into the outer thigh*); and (3) prepackaged nasal spray (NARCAN, *nasal spray, a prefilled, needle-free device that requires no assembly and is sprayed into 1 nostril*) [49]. More information and instructions for the safe use of naloxone to reverse clinically significant opioid-induced respiratory depression can be found at https://www.drugabuse.gov/drug-topics/opioids/opioid-overdose-reversal-naloxone-narcan-evzio.

SUMMARY

Assessment and management of pediatric pain present a unique challenge and opportunity for the HCP. Consideration of all variables that may be contributing to the pain experience, guided by the biopsychosocial model, will inform decisions regarding appropriate interventions. Therapeutic interventions, including nonpharmacologic and pharmacologic strategies, may be used to relieve pain in this vulnerable population. Knowledge of the guiding principles of pain management and available interventions will reinforce the critical role of the HCP in the holistic care of children and their families.

CLINICS CARE POINTS

- Experience and perception of pain is personal, even in children.
- Utilizing a step-wise approach for assessment, diagnosis, and intervention is essential.
- Evaluation of pain should be multifaceted, ie bio-psycho-social, to support identification of appropriate interventions.
- Use of a validated tool is recommended to support comparison of initial and subsequent assessments.
- Pharmacologic approach, if appropriate, should be matched with pain acuity, severity, and pattern.
- Frequent re-assessment and adjustment is key as pain is managed.

Disclosure
The authors have no commercial or financial conflicts of interest.

References
[1] Carr DB. Pain is a public health problem – what does that mean and why should we care? Pain Med 2016;17(4):626–7.
[2] Institute of Medicine. Relieving pain in America: a blueprint for transforming prevention, care, education, and research. 2011. Available at: https://www.nap.edu/catalog/13172/relieving-pain-in-america-a-blueprint-for-transforming-prevention-care. Accessed August 30, 2020.
[3] Merskey H, Albe Fessard D, Bonica JJ, et al. Pain terms: a list with definitions and notes on usage. Recommended by the IASP subcommittee on taxonomy. Pain 1979;6:249–52.
[4] Raja SN, Carr DB, Cohen M. The revised International Association for the Study of Pain definition of pain: concepts, challenges, and compromises. Pain 2020; https://doi.org/10.1097/j.pain.0000000000001939.
[5] Gatchel RJ, Howard KJ. The biopsychosocial approach. Practical pain management. Available at: https://www.practicalpainmanagement.com/treatments/psychological/biopsychosocial-approach. Accessed August 30, 2020.
[6] Fillinim RB. Individual differences in pain: understanding the mosaic that makes pain personal. Pain 2017;158(Suppl 1):S11–8.
[7] Roditi D, Robinson ME. The role of psychological interventions in the management of patients with chronic pain. Psychol Res Behav Manag 2011;4:41–9.
[8] Dekkers W. Pain as a Subjective and Objective Phenomenon. In: Schramme T, Edwards S. Handbook of the Philosophy of Medicine. Springer, Dordrecht. https://doi.org/10.1007/978-94-017-8706-2_8-1.
[9] Hurley-Wallace A, Wood C, Franck LS, et al. Paediatric pain education for health care professionals. Pain Rep 2019;4(1):e701.

[10] Kolcaba's theory of comfort. 2016. Available at: https://nursing-theory.org/theories-and-models/kolcaba-theory-of-comfort.php. Accessed August 7, 2020.

[11] Wilson L, Kolcaba K. Practical application of comfort theory in the perianesthesia setting. J Perianesth Nurs 2004;19(3):164–73.

[12] U.S. Department of Health and Human Services. Pain management best practices inter-agency task force report: updates, gaps, inconsistencies, and recommendations. 2019. Available at: https://www.hhs.gov/ash/advisory-committees/pain/reports/index.html. Accessed August 10, 2020.

[13] Srouji R, Ratnapalan S, Schneeweiss S. Pain in children: assessment and nonpharmacolog-ical management. Int J Pediatr 2010; https://doi.org/10.1155/2010/474838.

[14] Manworren RCB, Stinson J. Pediatric pain measurement, assessment, and evaluation. Semin Pediatr Neurol 2016;23:189–200.

[15] Maxwell LG, Malavolta CP, Fraga MV. Assessment of pain in the neonate. Clin Perinatol 2013;40:457–69.

[16] Redmann AJ, Wang Y, Furstein J, et al. The use of the FLACC pain scale in pediatric patients undergoing adenotonsillectomy. Int J Pediatr Otorhinolaryngol 2017;92:115–8.

[17] Tsze DS, vonBaeyer CL, Pahalyants V, et al. Validity and reliability of the Verbal Numerical Rating Scale for children aged 4 to 17 years with acute pain. Ann Emerg Med 2018;71(6):691–702.

[18] WHO guidelines for the pharmacological and radiotherapeutic management of cancer pain in children and adolescents. Geneva (Switzerland): World Health Organization; 2018 License: CC BY-NC-SA 3.0 IGO.

[19] Vargas-Schaffer G. Is the WHO analgesic ladder still valid? Can Fam Physician 2010;56(6):514–7.

[20] Hospice National, Palliative Care Organization. Pediatric pain management strategies. 2017. Available at: https://www.nhpco.org/wp-content/uploads/2019/04/PALLIATI-VECARE_PediatricPainManagement.pdf. Accessed August 11, 2020.

[21] Tick H, Nielsen A, Pelletier KR, et al. Evidence-based nonpharmacologic strategies for comprehensive pain care: the Consortium Pain Task Force White Paper. Explore 2018;14(3):177–211.

[22] Vega E, Rivera G, Echevarria GC, et al. Interventional procedures in children and adoles-cents with chronic non-cancer pain as part of a multidisciplinary pain management pro-gram. Paediatr Anaesth 2018;28(11):999–1006.

[23] Shah RD, Cappiello D, Suresh S. Interventional procedures for chronic pain in children and adolescents: a review of current evidence. Pain Pract 2016;16(3):359–69.

[24] Short G, Page G, Birnbaum C. Nonpharmacologic techniques to assist in pediatric pain management. Clin Pediatr Emerg Med 2017;18(4):256–60.

[25] McClafferty H, Vohra S, Bialey M, et al. Pediatric integrative medicine. Pediatrics 2017;140(3):e20171961.

[26] Tauben D. Nonopioid medications for pain. Phys Med Rehabil Clin N Am 2015;26:219–48.

[27] Pathan H, Williams J. Basic opioid pharmacology: an update. Br J Pain 2012;6(1):11–6.

[28] Kanabar DJ. A clinical and safety review of paracetamol and ibuprofen in children. Inflam-mopharmacology 2017;25(1):1–9.

[29] Brune K, Patrignani P. New insights into the use of currently available non-steroidal anti-in-flammatory drugs. J Pain Res 2015;8:105–18.

[30] Abramson S, Weissman G. The mechanisms of action of nonsteroidal anti-inflammatory drugs. Clin Exp Rheumatol 1989;7(Supp3):S163–70.

[31] Meade EA, Smith WL, DeWitt DL. Differential inhibition of prostaglandin endoperoxide syn-thase (cyclooxygenase) isoenzymes by aspirin and other non-steroidal anti-inflammatory drugs. J Biol Chem 1993;268(9):6610–4.

[32] Walsh P, Rothenberg SJ, Bang H. Safety of ibuprofen in infants younger than six months: a retrospective cohort study. PLoS One 2018;13(6):e0199493.

[33] Risser A, Donovan D, Heintzman J, et al. NSAID prescribing precautions. Am Fam Physician 2009;80(12):1371–8.

[34] Martino M, Chiarugi A, Boner A, et al. Working towards an appropriate use of ibuprofen in children: an evidence-based appraisal. Drugs 2017;77(12):1295–311.

[35] Lesko SM, Mitchell AA. An assessment of the safety of pediatric ibuprofen. A practitioner-based randomized clinical trial. JAMA 1995;273(12):929–33.

[36] O'Donnell FT, Rosen KR. Pediatric pain management: a review. Mo Med 2014;111(3):231–7.

[37] Botting RM. Mechanism of action of acetaminophen: is there a cyclooxygenase 3? Clin Infect Dis 2000;31(Suppl 5):S202–10.

[38] Lexicomp. Acetaminophen. Hudson (OH): Lexicomp; 2020.

[39] Sullivan D, Lyons M, Montgomery R, et al. Exploring opioid-sparing multimodal analgesia options in trauma: a nursing perspective. J Trauma Nurs 2016;23(6):361–75.

[40] Friedrichsdorf SJ, Kang EI. The management of pain in children with life-limiting illnesses. Pediatr Clin North Am 2007;54(5):645–72.

[41] Food and Drug Association. FDA drug safety communication: FDA restricts use of prescription codeine pain and cough medicines and tramadol pain medicines in children; recommends against use in breastfeeding women. 2018. Available at: https://www.fda.gov/drugs/drug-safety-and-availability/fda-drug-safety-communication-fda-restricts-use-prescription-codeine-pain-and-cough-medicines-and. Accessed August 12, 2020.

[42] Tobias JD, Green TP, Cote CJ, AAP SECTION ON ANESTHESIOLOGY AND PAIN MEDICINE, AAP COMMITTEE ON DRUGS. Codeine: time to say "no". Pediatrics 2016; https://doi.org/10.1542/peds2016-2396.

[43] Feudtner C, Freedman J, Kang T, et al. Comparative effectiveness of senna to prevent problematic constipation in pediatric oncology patients receiving opioids: a multicenter study of clinically detailed administrative data. J Pain Symptom Manage 2014;48(2):272–80.

[44] Matron KL, Johnson PN. Advocacy Committee on behalf of Pediatric Pharmacy Advocacy Group. Opioid use in children. J Pediatr Pharmacol Ther 2019;24(1):72–5.

[45] Fearon P, Hotopf M. Relation between headache in childhood and physical and psychiatric symptoms in adulthood: national birth cohort study. Br Med J 2001;322:1145.

[46] Walker LS, Dengler-Crish CM, Rippel S, et al. Functional abdominal pain in childhood and adolescence increases risk for chronic pain in adulthood. PAIN 2010;150:568–72.

[47] Centers for Disease Control. Prescription drug monitoring programs (PDMPs). Available at: https://www.michigan.gov/documents/mdhhs/PDMPs_618273_7.pdf. Accessed August 8, 2020.

[48] Centers for Disease Control. CDC guideline for prescribing opioids for chronic pain. Available at: https://www.cdc.gov/drugoverdose/pdf/Guidelines_At-A-Glance-508.pdf. Accessed August 8, 2020.

[49] National Institutes of Health. Opioid overdose reversal with naloxone (Narcan, Evzio). 2020. Available at: https://www.drugabuse.gov/drug-topics/opioids/opioid-overdose-reversal-naloxone-narcan-evzio. Accessed August 12, 2020.

CPI Antony Rowe
Eastbourne, UK
May 20, 2021